MYOCARDIAL VIABILITY

Developments in
Cardiovascular Medicine

VOLUME 154

The titles published in this series are listed at the end of this volume.

Myocardial viability

Detection and clinical relevance

Edited by

ABDULMASSIH S. ISKANDRIAN
Clinical Professor of Medicine, University of Pennsylvania School of Medicine,
Philadelphia, Pennsylvania; Co-Director Philadelphia Heart Institute, Director,
Noninvasive Cardiac Imaging, Philadelphia Heart Institute, Presbyterian
Medical Center, Philadelphia, Pennsylvania, U.S.A

and

ERNST E. VAN DER WALL
Associate Professor of Cardiology, Department of Cardiology,
Director, Cardiovascular Imaging Laboratory,
University Hospital Leiden, Leiden, The Netherlands

Springer Science+Business Media, B.V.

Library of Congress Cataloging-in-Publication Data

Myocardial viability : detection and clinical relevance / edited by
    Abdulmassih S. Iskandrian and Ernst E.van der Wall.
        p.   cm. -- (Developments in cardiovascular medicine ; v. 154)
    Includes index.
    ISBN 978-94-010-4510-0   ISBN 978-94-011-1170-6 (eBook)
    DOI 10.1007/978-94-011-1170-6
    1. Myocardium--Pathophysiology.   I. Iskandrian, Abdulmassih S.,
    1941-   . II. Wall, E. van der. III. Series.
    [DNLM: 1. Myocardial Diseases--diagnosis. 2. Heart Function
    Tests. 3. Myocardial Diseases--physiopathology. 4. Myocardium-
    -pathology.   W1 DE997VME v. 154 1994 / WG 280 M9969 1994]
    RC685.M9M87 1994
    616.1'24--dc20
    DNLM/DLC
    for Library of Congress   94-13373

ISBN 978-94-010-4510-0

Printed on acid-free paper

Dedicated
to
Our Wives,

Greta P. Iskandrian and Barbara J.M. van der Wall

and our children

Basil	Hein
Susan and	Sake and
Kristen	Ernst Lucas

Contents

List of Contributors

STEVEN R. BERGMANN
  Cardiovascular Division, Washington University Medical Center, Box 8086,
  660 South Euclid Avenue, St. Louis, MO 63110-1093, U.S.A.

MITCHELL S. FINKEL
  Laboratory of Molecular Cardiology, Montefiore University Hospital,
  University of Pittsburgh, 3459 Fifth Avenue, Pittsburgh, PA 15213, U.S.A
  Co-authors: Carmine V. Oddis, Brack G. Hattler & Richard L. Simmons

AMI S. ISKANDRIAN
  Co-Director, Philadelphia Heart Institute, Presbyterian Medical Center,
  39th and Market Streets, Philadelphia, PA 19104, U.S.A.

LYNNE L. JOHNSON
  Division of Cardiology, ZRB-310, University of Alabama at Birmingham,
  703 South 19th Street, Birmingham, AL 35294, U.S.A.

SANJIV KAUL
  Cardiovascular Division, Box 158, University of Virginia, Charlottesville,
  VA 22908, U.S.A.

MORTON J. KERN
  Director, J.G. Mudd Cardiac Catheterization Laboratory, St. Louis
  University Hospital, 3635 Vista Avenue at Grand Blvd, Box 15250, St. Louis,
  MO 63110-0250, U.S.A.
  Co-author: Michael S. Flynn

PIERRE RIGO
  Nuclear Medicine Department, Centre Hospitalier Universitaire B.35, Sart-
  Tilman, B-4000 Liège, Belgium
  Co-authors: Therèse Benoit & Simon Braat

ERNST E. VAN DER WALL
  Department of Cardiology, University Hospital Leiden, Building 1, C5-P25,
  Rijnsburgerweg 10, 2333 AA Leiden, The Netherlands
  Co-author: Hubert W. Vliegen

EDNA H.G. VENNEKER
Department of Diagnostic Radiology and Nuclear Medicine, University Hospital Leiden, Building 1, C4-Q, Rijnsburgerweg 10, 2333 AA Leiden, The Netherlands
Co-authors: Berthe L.F. van Eck-Smit & Gerda L. van Rijk-Zwikker

1. Introduction

ABDULMASSIH S. ISKANDRIAN & ERNST E. VAN DER WALL

The assessment of myocardial viability has recently emerged as an area of immense research interest and clinical relevance. There are important differences in myocardial blood flow, metabolism, and function between viable and nonviable myocardium. From the clinical viewpoint, the most important concern is to differentiate reversible from irreversible myocardial dysfunction. This distinction has important implications in patient management. With the growing interest in this area the term 'viability' itself has been under scrutiny. We, therefore, envisioned the need for a book devoted entirely to 'myocardial viability' and are most fortunate to have been able to recruit the help of prominent authorities in their respective fields of expertise.

In Chapter 2, Drs. Finkel and associates discuss the pathophysiological changes in myocardial metabolism and blood flow during ischemia, stunning and hibernation. Depression of the left ventricular contractility is complex; animal data incriminate changes in adenosine triphosphate, contractile proteins, excitation/contraction coupling, oxygen-free radicals and calcium overloading as potential mechanisms. A novel hypothesis based on cytokines and nitric oxide provides a new insight into the pathogenesis of reversible myocardial depression. Cytokines are antigen-specific glycoproteins that are synthesized rapidly and released locally by immune cells.

In Chapter 3, Dr. Johnson discusses the thallium-201 kinetics, the principles involved in the reinjection and delayed imaging, and the importance of quantitative assessment. Dual isotope imaging using antimyosin antibody and thallium-201 may be useful to delineate the area of necrosis and viable myocardium, based on the presence of matched, mismatched and overlap patterns. The pros and cons of rest-redistribution imaging versus other approaches such as stress-redistribution-reinjection, stress-redistribution-delayed imaging, and stress-immediate reinjection imaging are also presented. Suffice it to say, if the main issue is related to assessment of myocardial viability, rest-redistribution thallium imaging may provide the necessary information. If additional information on ischemia is needed, stress imaging has to be added.

In Chapter 4, Drs. Rigo, Benoit, and Braat discuss the use of technetium-99m Sestamibi perfusion imaging in the assessment of myocardial viability. The term viability was redefined as reversible chronic dysfunction in jeopardized myocardium susceptible to recover normal function following restoration of blood flow. Quantitative assessment, gated imaging and simultaneous

A.S. Iskandrian and E.E. van der Wall (eds): Myocardial viability, 1–4.
© 1994 *Kluwer Academic Publishers.*

assessment of perfusion and function may be important. Further, modification of the imaging protocol may also be useful. For example, the use of nitroglycerin before the rest images may improve the detection of viability. The authors challenge the issue that technetium-99m Sestamibi is primarily a perfusion agent rather than a marker of viability such as thallium-201. To refine the definition of myocardial viability, the use of thresholds is advocated for each individual tracer in order to distinguish between lack of viability below a certain predefined threshold and presence of viability above that threshold. In this regard, technetium-99m Sestamibi could serve well as a viability tracer using adequate preset thresholds.

In Chapter 5, Dr. Bergmann discusses the use of positron emission tomography, generally regarded as the gold standard. The high sensitivity and specificity of positron emission tomography and its ability to quantitatively evaluate myocardial perfusion and metabolism using physiologically appropriate mathematical models has provided a template for the evaluation of perfusion and metabolic imaging to define viability. The concept of a perfusable tissue index for delineation of myocardial viability using labeled water may constitute a rapid and convenient approach if proven sensitive and specific after studying a large number of patients. Although initially promising as a metabolic tracer, carbon-11 palmitate is decreasingly used due to influence of arterial fatty acid concentration on extraction and kinetics of carbon-11 palmitate, and due to the observation of back diffusion of unaltered tracer. The use of fluorine-18 deoxyglucose appears more promising to assess myocardial viability under many circumstances. Mismatch of perfusion and metabolism denotes residual viability which has major therapeutical and prognostic implications. However, distinction of viable and nonviable myocardium is suboptimal with fluorine-18 deoxyglucose and, in addition, the tracer does not distinguish between aerobic and anaerobic metabolism. Most promising results have been observed with carbon-11 acetate which is a marker of oxidative metabolism optimally reflecting myocardial viability. Levels of metabolism delineated with carbon-11 acetate predicted recovery of function after revascularization. Single-photon metabolic tracers, such as iodine-123 labeled free fatty acids, appear useful as markers of viability although limited data are available. Further correlative studies will be necessary to define the ultimate role and utility of iodinated free fatty acids as markers of myocardial viability.

In Chapter 6, Dr. Kaul discusses the application of echocardiography. There are two main methods: first, assessment of myocardial thickening and wall motion and, second, assessment of microvascular flow using contrast echocardiography. The use of wall thickening is based on experimental and clinical data suggesting a linear correlation between thickening and myocardial blood flow. Myocardial thickening stops when the myocardial flow decreases to 30% of the normal flow. Myocardial thickening is more prominent in the endocardial than the epicardial layers of the myocardium. Although preservation of thickening denotes the presence of a small area of necrosis, the loss of thickening, however, does not preclude the presence of viable myocardium. Wall motion assessment is affected by the tethering effect and by translational movement due to respiration, and is sensitive to changes in the loading conditions. Therefore, assessment of thickening is probably preferable to wall motion. Dobutamine echocardiography examines the contractile reserve of the myocardium and may result in both worsening or improvement in function, depending on the presence or absence of a flow-limiting lesion in infarct artery. In patients with acute myocardial infarction after thrombolytic therapy, myocardial salvage prevents left ventricular dilation and infarct expansion because of the buttressing effect of the viable myocardium. It may very well be that the lack of dilation or infarct expansion are indirect evidences of viable myocardium. The dose of dobutamine to detect enhancement of wall thickening depends on the extent of myocardial necrosis and the presence or absence of flow-limiting lesion and, therefore, a low dose may not be ideal for all patients. Furthermore, in hibernating myocardium where the flow is reduced at rest, dobutamine may cause worsening of function. Improvement is probably more common with stunned than hibernating myocardium. More studies are needed to assess the use of dobutamine echocardiography in hibernating myocardium. Contrast echocardiography involves injection of microbubbles of air (4–6 μ) that provide opacification of the myocardium because these bubbles remain entirely within the intravascular space and reflect the status of the microvascular perfusion in that region. Clinical studies have shown that, in patients with acute myocardial infarction, the extent of the collateral bed supplied by collateral flow (depicted by contrast echocardiography) is a good predictor of functional recovery after coronary angioplasty.

In Chapter 7, Drs. Van der Wall and Vliegen discuss the use of magnetic resonance imaging. The unique features of magnetic resonance imaging include good anatomical and temporal resolution, three-dimensional capabilities, easy reproducibility, and unlimited field of view and the possibility of *in vivo* measurement of myocardial biochemistry. To date, these techniques are only sparsely used for this purpose, probably because of long scanning times and relatively high costs of the equipment. Recent developments, like high speed subsecond imaging, will have significant impact on the time required for the study and may prove valuable in the detection of a wide range of pathophysiological entities such as flow, perfusion, wall motion and cardiac metabolism.

In Chapter 8, Drs. Kern and Flynn discusses the use of cardiac catheterization. It should be clear that coronary angiography is important for patient selection for revascularization purposes. Viability assessment in the catheterization laboratory is dependent on assessment of left ventricular function by contrast ventriculography using post-extrasystolic potentiation or nitroglycerin infusion. Hemodynamic variables are usually not useful in predicting viable myocardium. Caution, however, should be exercised in interpretation of wall motion on qualitative basis with these interventions because of translational and tethering effects discussed earlier. The centerline method of quantitative assessment of chordal shortening appears to be a more appropriate method.

Improvement in regional function in post-extrasystolic beat generally predicts improvement after revascularization. On the other hand, the lack of improvement does not preclude improvement with revascularization.

In Chapter 9, Drs. Venneker, van Eck-Smit, and van Rijk-Zwikker provide the cardiac surgeons' viewpoint about importance of viability in patients undergoing surgical revascularization. They report about complications and survival following coronary artery surgery. Furthermore, the value of preoperative assessment of myocardial viability by thallium scintigraphy and positron emission tomography using fluorine-18 deoxyglucose in predicting the functional recovery is discussed. Both methods are able to predict functional recovery in viable segments and, in addition, the absence of functional recovery in nonviable segments following coronary artery bypass surgery quite accurately. Therefore, assessment of myocardial viability may be useful to identify those patients in high risk groups such as patients with poor left ventricular function (EF <30%) who may benefit from coronary surgery. Furthermore, identification of viable myocardium is not necessary in patients with an EF > 30% because morbidity and mortality are acceptable and therefore the indication for coronary surgery will not change regardless of the presence of viability. Thallium-201 scintigraphy appears very useful in the assessment of graft patency after coronary bypass surgery.

Finally, in Chapter 10, we provide a summary and perspectives. The main issues addressed are the patients who need viability assessment, the optimum method to detect viability, and the factors that govern the recovery of left ventricular function after coronary revascularization.

This book has been developed for cardiologists, radiologists, nuclear medicine physicians, internists, basic scientists, cardiac surgeons and anesthesiologists and their trainees. Although this field is rapidly changing, we have, nevertheless, managed to include all relevant information through 1993 in this book. We would like to acknowledge the contributions of so many excellent investigators in this field who have stimulated the research and, in the process, have contributed to improving patient care.

We are most grateful for the support, understanding and patience of our wives and children. We would like also to thank Nettie Dekker from Kluwer Academic Publishers for her invaluable help, our secretaries Josette Costello and Anneke Van der Mey, for their efforts, and Jan Schoone from the Leiden University Library, for checking references and providing the index of the book.

2. Myocardial ischemia, stunning and hibernation: blood blow, metabolism and pathophysiology mechanism

MITCHELL S. FINKEL, CARMINE V. ODDIS,
BRACK G. HATTLER & RICHARD L. SIMMONS

Introduction

It was first shown in the opened chest dog model that ischemia followed by reperfusion was associated with a period of depressed myocardial contractility [1–4]. The clinical implications of these experimental observations were not fully appreciated until sophisticated imaging techniques enabled clinicians to non-invasively assess myocardial contractility and viability in patients [5, 6]. Quite surprisingly, it became increasingly apparent that a number of clinical conditions resulted in reversible depression of myocardial contractility. Reversible myocardial depression following reperfusion of ischemic myocardium was documented in patients following myocardial infarction, cardiopulmonary bypass, thrombolytic therapy and coronary angioplasty [5, 6]. This condition has been referred to as 'stunned' myocardium. Coronary artery bypass grafting (CABG) of chronically ischemic myocardium was also shown to result in improvement in the left ventricular ejection fraction in some patients [7, 8]. The term 'hibernating myocardium' has been adopted to refer to reversibly depressed chronically ischemic myocardium that remains viable but does not contract [9].

It has also recently been shown that sepsis can result in a transient period of reversible myocardial depression [10]. The relationship, if any, between 'stunned' and 'hibernating' myocardium and sepsis remains to be demonstrated. The basic mechanisms involved in sepsis-induced myocardial depression appear to be highly relevant to elucidating the mechanism(s) responsible for 'stunned' and 'hibernating' myocardium.

To understand the basic mechanisms responsible for reversible myocardial depression, it is necessary to appreciate how normal heart muscle contracts. Many review articles and books have been written on the basic mechanisms involved in muscle contraction [11–13]. Unfortunately, it is difficult to glean the clinically salient features of many of these lengthy documents. This chapter is an attempt to simplify and distill the critical principles of cardiovascular physiology that are directly relevant to understanding the mechanisms responsible for reversible myocardial depression.

A.S. Iskandrian and E.E. van der Wall (eds): Myocardial viability, 5–18.
© *1994 Kluwer Academic Publishers.*

Myocardial contractility

As a starting point, myocardial contractility can be viewed as regulated by one of three components: 1) calcium, 2) ATP, and 3) contractile proteins (Figure 2.1). Rapid changes in myocardial contractility presumably relate to changes at the level of intracellular ionized free-calcium in the cardiac myocyte [11–13]. Physiologic and pharmacologic manipulation of the ion channels responsible for increasing or decreasing contractility will be described in detail later.

Ca $^{2+}$ ATP

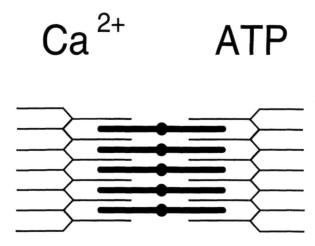

Figure 2.1. Schematic illustration of the three major components responsible for myocardial contractility. Ca^{++}, calcium refers to ionized free calcium in the cell; ATP, adenosine triphosphate refers to the metabolic energy in the cell; Contractile proteins.

ATP refers to the metabolic energy of the cell (Figure 2.2). The availability of oxygen during aerobic conditions allows 36 moles of ATP to be produced per mole of glucose [13]. Free fatty acids are the major metabolic substrate for ATP production in the well perfused myocardium [13, 14]. Anaerobic glycolysis that occurs during ischemia is far less efficient and produces only two moles of ATP per mole of glucose. PET scanning of chronically ischemic hibernating myocardium has shown an increase in glucose uptake [15, 16]. This presumably relates to the enhanced glycolytic activity of this viable but poorly contracting muscle. Studies of stunned myocardium have failed to consistently demonstrate significant changes in ATP levels following ischemia and reperfusion [17]. The role of ATP in either stunned or hibernating myocardium is not obvious. ATP levels do not appear to be sufficiently depressed during ischemia to adequately explain depression in myocardial contractility.

Alterations in contractile proteins alone are also unlikely to be responsible for reversible myocardial depression seen in stunned and hibernating myocardium (Figure 2.3). The affinity of contractile proteins for calcium may play a role in the initial depression of contractility associated with various ischemic syndromes [17–20]. Experimental studies have indicated that affinity

CARDIAC CELL

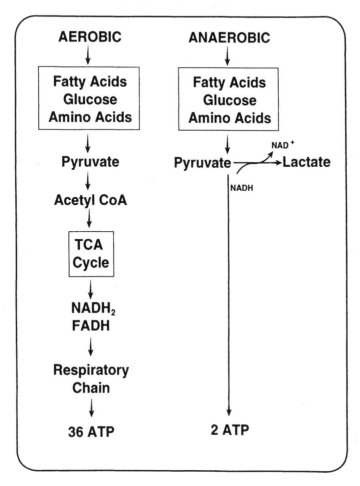

Figure 2.2. Illustration of the metabolic pathways for cellular ATP production in the cardiac cell. TCA, tricarboxylic acid cycle.

of contractile proteins for calcium may be altered by ischemia and reperfusion [20]. However, it is unlikely that profound reversible effects on inotropy are explicable solely on the basis of changes in the affinity of contractile proteins for calcium.

A more likely explanation for changes in myocardial contractility seen in stunned and hibernating myocardium should relate to alterations in excitation-contraction coupling (E-C coupling) (Figure 2.4). This term refers to the relationship between depolarization of the myocyte membrane and the resultant contraction [11]. This is a very complicated process that clearly involves the movement of calcium from outside the cell into the cell and back out again. The major regulators of the transsarcolemmal transport of calcium include the L-type sarcolemmal calcium channels, beta- and alpha-adrenergic receptors and

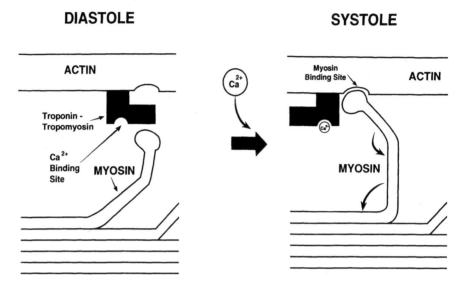

Figure 2.3. Illustration depicting myocardial contraction. The availability of calcium induces the conformational change in the troponin-tropomyosin complex that allows myosin and actin to interact.

receptor-operated calcium channels [11, 13, 21]. These membrane bound proteins all contribute to the influx of only a minute quantity of calcium from outside the cell into the myocyte. The small quantity of calcium that traverses the L-type calcium channel during membrane depolarization causes the release of the large reservoir of calcium stored in the sarcoplasmic reticulum (SR) through the SR calcium release channel [11, 22]. This large reservoir of calcium then interacts with tropomyosin to allow the actin and myosin filaments to overlap (Figure 2.3). This results in systolic myocardial contraction. Diastolic relaxation results with the resequestration of this large reservoir of calcium back into the sarcoplasmic reticulum through the SR calcium/ATPase [23–25]. The minute quantity of transsarcolemmal 'trigger' calcium is passed back out of the cell through the Na^+/Ca^{++} exchanger [11, 13].

Considerably more detail is known about the mechanisms by which autonomic receptors regulate calcium influx through the sarcolemma [11, 21, 26–33]. Beta adrenergic stimulation results in the association of a catalytic subunit of a G-protein coupled to the Beta-receptor. This stimulates the enzyme, adenylate cyclase, to convert ATP to cAMP [26–29]. Increasing cAMP production results in cAMP dependent phosphorylation of the L-type calcium channel [26–29]. Phosphorylation results in an increase in the probability for the open state of the channel. This translates into an increase in transsarcolemmal calcium influx during phase 2 (i.e. the plateau phase) of the action potential. Alpha adrenergic receptor stimulation results in the phospholipase C-mediated breakdown of phosphatidylcholine to inositol triphosphate (IP_3) and diacyl glycerol (DAG) [30–33]. These second messengers further enhance mobilization of both transsarcolemmal calcium influx and SR calcium efflux.

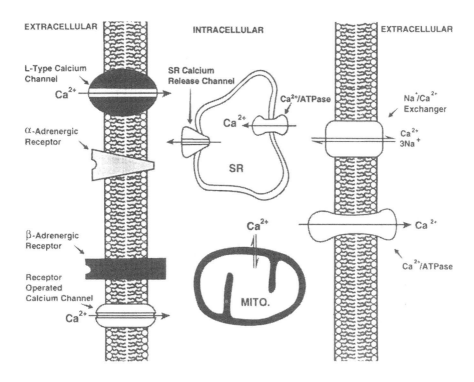

Figure 2.4. Illustration of the movement of calcium extracellularly to trigger intracellular release of calcium followed by extrusion of calcium back into the extracellular space. Calcium enters the myocyte through L-type calcium channels that are modulated by adrenergic receptors. This small quantity of calcium triggers the release of the large reservoir of intracellular calcium stored in the SR (sarcoplasmic reticulum) by activation of the SR calcium release channel. Calcium is resequestered into the SR by the SR calcium/ATPase. Calcium also shuttles across the mitochondria. Calcium is extruded from the cell largely through the Na^+/Ca^{++} exchanger and the sarcolemmal calcium ATPase.

The mechanism by which transsarcolemmal calcium activates the release of SR calcium is not completely understood. It does appear to involve an allosteric conformational change in the SR release channel caused by the binding of calcium to a specific site (Figure 2.5) [22]. It has recently been shown that sulfhydryl reagents also significantly alter the characteristics of the SR calcium release channel [34–38]. The oxidation or reduction of free sulfhydryls on the SR calcium release channel appear to be physiologically important regulators of SR calcium release [34–38].

Hypotheses

Several hypotheses have been proposed to explain the myocardial depression seen in both stunned and hibernating myocardium:

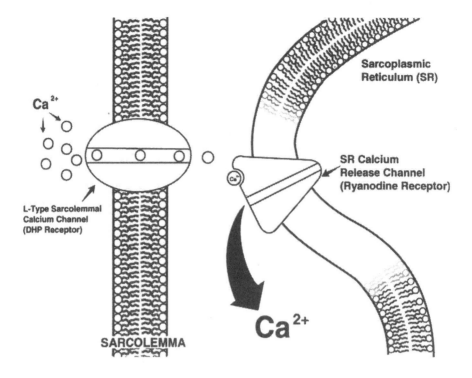

Figure 2.5. Illustration of the calcium-induced calcium release mechanism for E-C coupling in the cardiac myocyte. A small quantity of extracellular calcium passes through the L-type sarcolemmal calcium channel which triggers the release of the large reservoir of SR calcium through activation of the SR calcium release channel. DHP, dihydropyridine.

1. Oxygen free radicals [39–44]
2. Calcium overload [17]
3. E-C coupling [34, 35, 57]
4. Depressed ATP levels [63, 64]
5. White blood cells (65–70]
6. Nitric Oxide [71, 91]
7. Cytokines [71, 75]

A number of observations have been made in a variety of animal models and clinical conditions demonstrating the elaboration of reactive oxygen intermediates (oxygen-free radicals) in reperfused myocardium [39–51]. This has led many investigators to believe that oxygen-free radicals are responsible for reperfusion injury and cell death. Others have extended this view to include the reversible myocardial depression (stunned myocardium) also seen in association with the presence of oxygen-free radicals [40, 47]. Efforts to prevent the elaboration of oxygen-free radicals produced conflicting results [40, 41, 45, 47, 49–51]. This has shed some doubt on the pathogenetic significance of the presence of oxygen free radicals in reperfused myocardium:

Other investigators have focused their attention on the possible role of calcium overload in depressing myocardial contractility [52-56]. Interestingly, investigators have shown that the use of calcium channel blockers improves the survival of reperfused myocardium in animal models [52-56].

Some investigators have explored the role of alterations in excitation-contraction coupling as a cause of reversible myocardial dysfunction [57, 34, 35]. This hypothesis proposes that a defect in SR calcium release is responsible for either stunned or hibernating myocardium.

Still other investigators have implicated defective ATP utilization as a possible mechanism for myocardial depression [58-61]. However, several studies have indicated that ATP levels are adequate to sustain normal contractility following ischemia-reperfusion [62-64]. The availability of *in vivo* NMR spectroscopy has provided compelling evidence against a defect in metabolic energy production or utilization as a mechanism for reversible myocardial dysfunction [17, 62].

A very interesting series of studies were conducted suggesting that white blood cells contribute in some way to reperfusion injury and stunning [65-70]. Depletion of neutrophils prior to ischemia and reperfusion resulted in enhancement in the recovery of post-ischemic functioning in a dog model [65-70]. These findings were interpreted to mean that white blood cells are either a source of oxygen-free radicals or cause microvascular plugging and further ischemic damage.

Cytokines and nitric oxide

We and others have recently provided compelling evidence for the regulation of myocardial function by cytokines and nitric oxide (NO) [71-75]. These discoveries provide the basis for a novel hypothesis of the pathogenesis of the reversible myocardial depression seen clinically in septic and ischemic patients.

Nitric oxide is formed from the oxidation of one of the two chemically equivalent quanidino nitrogens of L-arginine by NO synthase [76-78]. Arginine analogues such as L-NMMA block the production of NO by competitively inhibiting NO synthase enzyme activity [79]. The addition of L-arginine can overcome this inhibition [79]. NO has been shown to have a variety of effects on cells, including raising cGMP levels by activating soluble guanylate cyclase [80].

Cytokines are antigen-nonspecific glycoproteins that are synthesized rapidly and released locally by immune cells [81]. Interleukins 1, 2, 6 and TNF (Tumor Necrosis Factor) are cytokines that are produced by immune cells in response to challenge or injury [81]. Interleukin (IL)-2 administration to cancer patients elicits reversible hemodynamic changes similar to those seen in shock due to gram-negative bacterial sepsis [82-85]. Patients develop sinus tachycardia, decreased mean arterial pressure, increased cardiac index, decreased systemic vascular resistance and a fall in left ventricular ejection fraction.

These hemodynamic effects of gram-negative bacteria have been attributed to endotoxin (lipopolysaccharide-LPS) in the bacterial membrane [86, 87]. LPS has recently been shown to mediate effects through stimulation of mononuclear phagocytes [86, 87]. Of the variety of mediators released by these cells, TNF, IL-1, and IL-6 appear to play a pivotal role in mediating the hemodynamic effects of gram-negative sepsis and shock. IL-1, TNF, and LPS have been demonstrated to cause hypotension [88]. Plasma IL-6 levels have been found to be increased 7,500 times the normal level in septic patients [89]. Our laboratory investigated possible immediate, direct effects and mechanisms of action of these cytokines on the heart [71].

TNF-α, IL-6, and IL-2 all reversibly depressed contractility of isolated left ventricular papillary muscles [71]. The NO synthase inhibitor, L-NMMA, blocked these negative inotropic effects. L-Arginine reversed the inhibition by L-NMMA. These results suggested that the direct negative inotropic effects of cytokines on the heart could be mediated through activation of a myocardial nitric oxide synthase.

Recently, it was demonstrated that these inflammatory cytokines reduced the positive inotropic response of isolated cardiac myocytes to the β-adrenergic agonist, isoproterenol, through a mechanism also possibly involving NO [72]. TNF and IL-1 have also been shown to uncouple agonist-occupied receptors from adenylate cyclase in isolated cardiac myocytes [73]. These findings implicate β-receptor or guanine nucleotide binding protein function in the direct of indirect action of cytokines on the heart. This is consistent with a cGMP-mediated effect of NO on myocardial contractility.

Cytokines have also been demonstrated to regulate each other's effects on the heart. Transforming growth factor (TGF) $-\beta$ has been shown to antagonize the chronotropic effects of IL-1 on isolated neonatal cardiac myocytes [74]. These effects are also consistent with a cGMP-mediated mechanism of action of NO on myocardial chronotropy. It is unknown whether the inotropic and chronotropic effects of cytokines are mediated through the regulation of a common ion channel. The regulation of the sarcolemmal L-type calcium channel could explain both the inotropic and chronotropic effects of cytokines on the heart.

In another study conducted in our laboratory, elevated levels of IL-6 were detected in patients immediately following aortocoronary bypass grafting [75]. These same concentrations of IL-6 were also shown by us to reversibly depress contractility in human cardiac tissue. Serum IL-6 levels have also recently been reported to be elevated in patients following myocardial infarction [90]. From these observations, it is intriguing to speculate that IL-6 could contribute to the transient myocardial depression, 'stunning', that is known to occur following cardiopulmonary bypass and myocardial infarction.

We further explored the potential role for NO in post-CABG myocardial stunning by assaying for its stable end-products, NO_2 (nitrite), and NO_3 (nitrate) [91]. Coronary sinus nitrite and nitrate levels were increased 10-fold in patients following coronary artery bypass surgery. In addition, NO synthase enzyme activity was increased 3-fold in pectinate muscles from these patients following the same surgery. These elevated levels of NO products were temporally associated with post-operative myocardial stunning. Taken together, our findings support a cytokine-stimulated, NO-mediated mechanism for myocardial stunning following cardiopulmonary bypass.

Hibernating myocardium

There is currently no evidence to support a cytokine-nitric oxide mediated mechanism for the reversible myocardial depression seen in chronic ischemia (hibernating myocardium). However, our previous discussion regarding E-C coupling in the heart is very relevant to understanding the most likely mechanisms that are common to both stunning and hibernating. Regardless of the stimulus, reversible myocardial depression is most likely related to alterations in E-C coupling in the heart. Evidence is accumulating to support a cytokine-nitric oxide mediated alteration in E-C coupling in reversible myocardial dysfunction seen in sepsis and acute ischemia [10, 92]. A significant portion of this work has been done in animal models, which has provided important insights relevant to these clinical conditions. Animal models for hibernating myocardium are not as well described. This has certainly impacted on our understanding of the basic mechanisms responsible for hibernating myocardium in patients.

The cardiomyopathic Syrian hamster may ultimately prove to be a relevant model for hibernating myocardium in patients [93–100]. This animal has a genetic defect that results in calcium overload and premature death from congestive heart failure [97, 98]. Interestingly, considerable evidence exists that these animals are chronically ischemic on the basis of microvascular spasm [99, 100]. We proposed that chronic ischemia results in reversible myocardial depression in this animal model through an effect on E-C coupling [34, 35, 93]. We have provided compelling evidence for the existence of such a defect in sulfhydryl gating of the SR release channel in the myopathic hamster [34, 35, 93–95]. Chronic ischemia in patients may similarly cause sufficient depletion of ATP to alter the myocyte redox potential. Defective coupling between the sarcolemmal L-type calcium channel and the SR calcium release channel would result.

Summary

Recent advances in imaging techniques and therapeutic interventions have clearly demonstrated the importance of reversible myocardial dysfunction in patients with acute and chronic ischemic syndromes. It is also clear that a number of other clinical conditions such as sepsis are also associated with reversible myocardial depression. A better understanding of the basic mechanisms involved in normal myocardial contractility will undoubtedly play an essential role in future efforts to modify these clinical states. New discoveries regarding novel regulators of myocardial contractility may provide entirely new approaches to understanding the pathophysiologic mechanisms responsible for reversible myocardial depression. The rapid testing and application of these new physiologic concepts will be possible largely as a result of the highly sophisticated imaging techniques currently available.

Acknowledgements

This research was supported by awards from the American Heart Association, Western Pennsylvania Affiliate; The Sarah and David Weiss Cardiovascular Research Fellowship and the National Institutes of Health, Grant #GM-37753. The authors thank Mrs. Cynthia McQuillis for her assistance in the preparation of this manuscript.

References

1. Heyndrickx GR, Millard RW, McRitchie RJ, Maroko PR, Vatner SF. Regional myocardial functional and electrophysiological alterations after brief coronary occlusion in conscious dog. J Clin Invest 1975; 56: 978–85.
2. Ellis SG, Henschke CI, Sandor T, Wynne J, Braunwald E, Kloner RA. Time course of functional and biochemical recovery of myocardium salvaged by reperfusion. J Am Coll Cardiol 1983; 1: 1047–55.
3. Sayten JJ, Peirce G, Katcher AH, Sheldon WF. Correlation of intramyocardial electrocardiograms with polarographic oxygen and contractility in the nonischemic and regionally ischemic left ventricle. Circ Res 1961; 9: 1268–79.
4. Charlat ML, O'Neill PG, Hartley CJ, Roberts R, Bolli R. Prolonged abnormalities of left ventricular diastolic wall thinning in the 'stunned' myocardium in conscious dogs: Time course and relation to systolic function. J Am Coll Cardiol 1989; 13: 185–94.
5. Braunwald E, Kloner RA. The stunned myocardium: Prolonged, postischemic ventricular dysfunction. Circulation 1982; 66: 1146–9.
6. Dilsizian V, Bonow RO. Current diagnostic techniques of assessing myocardial viability in patients with hibernating and stunned myocardium. Circulation 1993; 1: 1–20.
7. Matsuzaki M, Gallagher KP, Kemper WS, White F, Ross J Jr. Sustained regional dysfunction produced by prolonged coronary stenosis: Gradual recovery after reperfusion. Circulation 1983; 68: 170–82.
8. Fedele FA, Gerwitz H, Capone RJ, Sharaf B, Most AS. Metabolic response to prolonged reduction of myocardial blood flow distal to a severe coronary artery stenosis. Circulation 1988; 78: 729–35.
9. Rahimtoola SH. The hibernating myocardium. Am Heart J 1989; 117: 211–21.
10. Parrillo JE. Pathogenetic mechanisms of septic shock. N Engl J Med 1993; 328: 1471–7.
11. Bers DM. Excitation-Contraction Coupling and Cardiac Contractile Force. Dordrecht, The Netherlands: Kluwer Academic Publishers 1991; 119–48.
12. Zot AS, Potter JD. Structural aspects of troponin-tropomyosin regulation of skeletal muscle contraction. Annu Rev Biophys Biophys Chem 1987; 16: 535–59.
13. Katz AM. Physiology of the Heart. 2nd ed. New York: Raven Press 1992.
14. Camici P, Marraccini P, Lorenzoni R, Ferrannini E, Buzzigoli G, Marzilli M *et al.* Metabolic markers of stress-induced myocardial ischemia. Circulation 1991; 83 (5 Suppl): III8–13.

15. Mody FV, Brunken RC, Stevenson LW, Nienaber CA, Phelps ME, Schelbert HR. Differentiating cardiomyopathy of coronary artery disease from nonischemic dilated cardiomyopathy utilizing positron emission tomography. J Am Coll Cardiol 1991; 17: 373–83.
16. Fudo T, Kambara H, Hashimoto T, Hayashi M, Nohara R, Tamaki N *et al.* F-18 deoxyglucose and stress N-13 ammonia positron emission tomography in anterior wall healed myocardial infarction. Am J Cardiol 1988; 61: 1191–7.
17. Marban E. Myocardial stunning and hibernation. The physiology behind the colloquialisms. Circulation 1991; 83: 681–8.
18. Fabiato A, Fabiato F. Effects of pH on the myofilaments and the sarcoplasmic reticulum of skinned cells from cardiac and skeletal muscles. J Physiol (Lond) 1978; 276: 233–55.
19. Kentish JC. The effects of inorganic phosphate and creatine phosphate on force production in skinned muscles from rat ventricle. J Physiol (Lond) 1986; 370: 585–604.
20. Marban E, Kusuoka H. Maximal Ca^{2+}-activated force and myofilament Ca^{2+} sensitivity in intact mammalian hearts. Differential effects of inorganic phosphate and hydrogen. Gen Physiol 1987; 90: 609–23.
21. Brown AM, Birnbaumer L. Direct G protein gating of ion channels. Am J Physiol 1988; 254: H401–10.
22. Fabiato A, Fabiato F. Calcium induced release of calcium from the sarcoplasmic reticulum of skinned cells from adult human, dog, cat, rabbit, rat and frog hearts and from fetal and newborn rat ventricles. Ann N Y Acad Sci 1978; 307: 491–522.
23. Ikemoto N. Structure and function of the calcium pump protein of sarcoplasmic reticulum. Annu Rev Physiol 1982; 44: 297–317.
24. Hasselbach W, Oetliker H. Energetics and electrogenicity of the sarcoplasmic reticulum calcium pump. Annu Rev Physiol 1983; 45: 325–39.
25. Tanford C. Mechanisms of free energy coupling in active transport. Annu Rev Biochem 1983; 52: 379–409.
26. Sperelakis N, Schneider JA. A metabolic control mechanism for calcium ion influx that may protect the ventricular myocardial cell. Am J Cardiol 1976; 37: 1079–85.
27. Reuter H, Scholz H. The regulation of the calcium conductance of cardiac muscle by adrenaline. J Physiol (Lond) 1977; 264: 49–62.
28. Hartzell HC. Regulation of cardiac ion channels by catecholamines, acetylcholine and second messenger systems. Prog Biophys Mol Biol 1988; 52: 165–247.
29. Hosey MM, Lazdunski M. Calcium channels: Molecular pharmacology, structure and regulation. J Membr Biol 1988; 104: 81–105.
30. Brown JH, Jones LG. Phosphoinositide metabolism in the heart. In Putney JW Jr (ed): Phosphoinositides and receptor mechanisms. New York: Alan R. Liss 1986; 245–70.
31. Poggioli J, Sulpice JC, Vassort G. Inositol phosphate production following alpha 1-adrenergic, muscarinic, or electrical stimulation in isolated rat heart. FEBS Lett 1986; 206: 292–8.
32. Jones LG, Goldstein D, Brown JH. Guanine nucleotide-dependent inositol triphosphate formation in chick heart cells. Circ Res 1988; 62: 299–305.
33. Scholz J, Schaefer B, Schmitz W, Scholz H, Steinfath M, Lohse M *et al.* Alpha-1 adrenoreceptor-mediated positive inotropic effect and inositol triphosphate increase in mammalian heart. J Pharmacol Exp Ther 1988; 245: 327–35.
34. Finkel MS, Shen L, Oddis CV, Romeo RC, Salama G. Positive inotropic effect of acetylcysteine in the cardiomyopathic Syrian hamster. J Cardiovasc Pharmacol 1993; 21: 29–34.
35. Finkel MS, Shen L, Oddis CV, Srivastava R, Salama G. Defective sulfhydryl gating of the SR calcium release channel in the cardiomyopathic Syrian hamster. Am J Phys 1994 In press.
36. Abramson JJ, Salama G. Regulation of the sarcoplasmic reticulum calcium permeability by sulfhydryl oxidation and reduction. J Membr Sci 1987; 33: 241–8.
37. Abramson JJ, Trimm JL, Weden L, Salama G. Heavy metals induce rapid calcium release from sarcoplasmic reticulum vesicles isolated from skeletal muscle. Proc Natl Acad Sci USA 1983; 80: 1526–30.
38. Prabhu SD, Salama G. The heavy metal ions Ag^+ and Hg^{2+} trigger calcium release from cardiac sarcoplasmic reticulum. Arch Biochem Biophys 1990; 277: 47–55.

39. Ambrosio G, Weisfeldt ML, Jacobus WE, Flaherty JT. Evidence for a reversible oxygen radical-mediated component of reperfusion injury: Reduction by recombinant human superoxide dismutase administered at the time of reflow. Circulation 1987; 75: 282–91.
40. Bolli R, Jeroudi MO, Patel BS, Aruoma OI, Halliwell B, Lai EK *et al*. Marked reduction of free radical generation and contractile dysfunction by antioxidant therapy begun at the time of reperfusion. Evidence that myocardial 'stunning' is a manifestation of reperfusion injury. Circ Res 1989; 65: 607–22.
41. Mehta JL, Nichols WW, Donnelly WH, Lawson DL, Thompson L, ter Riet M *et al*. Protection by superoxide dismutase from myocardial dysfunction and attenuation of vasodilator reserve after coronary occlusion and reperfusion in dog. Circ Res 1989; 65: 1283–95.
42. Kloner RA, Przyklenk K, Whittaker P. Deleterious effects of oxygen radicals in ischemia/reperfusion. Resolved and unresolved issues. Circulation 1989; 80: 1115–27.
43. Cohen MV. Free radicals in ischemic and reperfusion myocardial injury: Is this the time for clinical trials? Ann Intern Med 1989; 111: 918–31.
44. Kaneko M, Beamish RE, Dhalla NS. Depression of heart sarcolemmal Ca^{2+}-pump activity by oxygen free radicals. Am J Physiol 1989; 256: H368–74.
45. van der Kraaij AM, van Eijk HG, Koster JF. Prevention of postischemic cardiac injury by the orally active iron chelator 1,2-dimethyl-3-hydroxy-4-pyridone (L1) and the antioxidant (+)-cyanidanol-3. Circulation 1989; 80: 158–64.
46. Pallandi RT, Perry MA, Campbell TH. Proarrhythmic effects of an oxygen-derived free radical generating system on action potentials recorded from guinea pig ventricular myocardium: A possible cause of reperfusion-induced arrhythmias. Circ Res 1987; 61: 50–4.
47. Bolli R, Zhu WX, Hartley CJ, Michael LH, Repine JE, Hess ML *et al*. Attenuation of dysfunction in the postischemic 'stunned' myocardium by dimethylthiourea. Circulation 1987; 76: 458–68.
48. Engler R, Gilpin E. Can superoxide dismutase alter myocardial infarct size? Circulation 1989; 79: 1137–42.
49. Naslund U, Haggmark S, Johansson G, Marklund SL, Reiz S. Limitation of myocardial infarct size by superoxide dismutase as an adjunct to reperfusion after different durations of coronary occlusion in the pig. Circ Res 1990; 66: 1294–301.
50. Holzgrefe HH, Gibson JK. Beneficial effects of oxypurinol pretreatment in stunned, reperfused canine myocardium. Cardiovasc Res 1989; 23: 340–50.
51. Williams RE, Zweier JL, Flaherty JT. Treatment with deferoxamine during ischemia improves functional and metabolic recovery and reduces reperfusion-induced oxygen radical generation in rabbit hearts. Circulation 1991; 83: 1006–14.
52. Campbell CA, Kloner RA, Alker KJ, Braunwald E. Effect of verapamil on infarct size in dogs subjected to coronary artery occlusion with transient reperfusion. J Am Coll Cardiol 1986; 8: 1169–74.
53. Henry PD, Shuchleib R, Davis J, Weiss ES, Sobel BE. Myocardial contracture and accumulation of mitochondrial calcium in ischemic rabbit heart. Am J Physiol 1977; 233: H677–84.
54. DeBoer LW, Strauss HW, Kloner RA, Rude RE, Davis RF, Maroko PR *et al*. Autoradiographic method for measuring the ischemic myocardium at risk: Effects of verapamil on infarct size after experimental coronary artery occlusion. Proc Natl Acad Sci USA 1980; 77: 6119–23.
55. Nayler WG, Panagiotopoulos S, Elz JS, Sturrock WJ. Fundamental mechanisms of action of calcium antagonists in myocardial ischemia. Am J Cardiol 1987; 59: 75B–83B.
56. Kloner RA, Braunwald E. Effects of calcium antagonists on infarcting myocardium. Am J Cardiol 1987; 59: 84B–94B.
57. Stern MD, Silverman HS, Houser SR, Josephson RA, Capogrossi MC, Nichols CG *et al*. Anoxic contractile failure in rat heart myocytes is caused by failure of intracellular calcium release due to alteration of the action potential. Proc Natl Acad Sci USA 1988; 85: 6954–8.
58. Katz AM. The early 'pump' failure of the ischemic heart. Am J Med 1969; 47: 497–502.
59. Kubler W, Spieckermann PG. Regulation of glycolysis in the ischemic and the anoxic myocardium. J Mol Cell Cardiol 1970; 1: 351–77.

60. Reibel DK, Rovetto MJ. Myocardial ATP synthesis and mechanical function following oxygen deficiency. Am J Physiol 1978; 234: H620–4.
61. Vary TC, Angelakos ET, Schaffer SW. Relationship between adenine nucleotide metabolism and irreversible ischemic tissue damage in isolated perfused rat heart. Circ Res 1979; 45: 218–25.
62. Kusuoka H, Porterfield JK, Weisman HF, Weisfeldt ML, Marban E. Pathophysiology and pathogenesis of stunned myocardium. Depressed Ca^{2+}-activation as a consequence of reperfusion-induced cellular calcium overload in ferret hearts. J Clin Invest 1987; 79: 950–61.
63. Neely JR, Grotyohann LW. Role of glycolytic products in damage to ischemic myocardium. Dissociation of adenosine and triphosphate levels and recovery of function of reperfused ischemic hearts. Circ Res 1984; 55: 816–24.
64. Taegtmeyer H, Roberts AF, Raine AE. Energy metabolism in reperfused heart muscle: Metabolic correlates to return of function. J Am Coll Cardiol 1985; 6: 864–70.
65. Engler R, Covell JW. Granulocytes cause reperfusion ventricular dysfunction after 15-minute ischemia in the dog. Circ Res 1987; 61: 20–8.
66. Verrier ED, Shen I. Potential role of neutrophil anti-adhesion therapy in myocardial stunning, myocardial infarction, and organ dysfunction after cardiopulmonary bypass. J Card Surg 1993; 8 (2 Suppl): 309–12.
67. Westlin W, Mullane KM. Alleviation of myocardial stunning by leukocyte and platelet depletion. Circulation 1989; 80: 1828–36.
68. O'Neill PG, Charlat ML, Michael LH, Roberts R, Bolli R. Influence of neutrophil depletion on myocardial function and flow after reversible ischemia. Am J Physiol 1989; 256: H341–51.
69. Simpson PJ, Todd RF 3d, Fantone JC, Mickelson JK, Griffin JD, Luchesi BR. Reduction of experimental canine myocardial reperfusion injury by a monoclonal antibody (anti-Mo1, anti-CD11b) that inhibits leukocyte adhesion. J Clin Invest 1988; 81: 624–9.
70. Byrne JG, Appleyard RF, Lee CC, Couper GS, Scholl FG, Laurence AG et al. Controlled reperfusion of the regionally ischemic myocardium with leukocyte-depleted blood reduces stunning, the no-reflow phenomenon, and infarct size. J Thorac Cardiovasc Surg 1992; 103: 66–71; discussion 71–2.
71. Finkel MS, Oddis CV, Jacobs TD, Watkins SC, Hattler BG, Simmons RL. Negative inotropic effects of cytokines on the heart mediated by nitric oxide. Science 1992; 257: 387–9.
72. Balligand JL, Ungureanu D, Kelly RA, Kobzik L, Pimental D, Michel T et al. Abnormal contractile function due to induction of nitric oxide synthesis in rat cardiac myocytes follows exposure to activated macrophage-conditioned medium. J Clin Invest 1993; 91: 2314–9.
73. Gulick T, Chung MK, Peiper SJ, Lange LG, Schreiner GF. Interleukin 1 and tumor necrosis factor inhibit cardiac myocytes beta-adrenergic responsiveness. Proc Natl Acad Sci USA 1989; 86: 6753–7.
74. Roberts AB, Roche NS, Winokur TS, Burmester JK, Sporn MB. Role of transforming growth factor-beta in maintenance of function of cultured neonatal cardiac myocytes. Autocrine action and reversal of damaging effects of interleukin-1. J Clin Invest 1992; 90: 2056–62.
75. Finkel MS, Hoffman RA, Shen L, Oddis CV, Simmons RL, Hattler BG. Interleukin-6 (IL-6) as a mediator of stunned myocardium. Am J Cardiol 1993; 71: 1231–2.
76. Ignarro LJ, Buga GM, Wood KS, Byrns RE, Chaudhuri G. Endothelium-derived relaxing factor produced and released from artery and vein is nitric oxide. Proc Natl Acad Sci USA 1987; 84: 9265–9.
77. Palmer RM, Ferrige AG, Moncada S. Nitric oxide release accounts for the biological activity of endothelium-derived relaxing factor. Nature 1987; 327: 524–6.
78. Palmer RM, Ashton DS, Moncada S. Vascular endothelial cells synthesize nitric oxide from L-arginine. Nature 1988; 333: 664–6.
79. Dinerman JL, Lowenstein CJ, Snyder SH. Molecular mechanisms of nitric oxide regulation. Potential relevance to cardiovascular disease. Circ Res 1993; 73: 217–22.
80. Lowenstein CJ, Snyder SH. Nitric oxide, a novel biologic messenger. Cell 1992; 70: 705–7.
81. Abbas AK, Lichtman AH, Pober JS. Cellular and Molecular Immunology. Philadelphia: Saunders 1991; 226–43.

82. Zeilender S, David D, Fairman RP, Glauser FL. Inotropic and vasoactive drug treatment of interleukin 2 induced hypotension in sheep. Cancer Res 1989; 49: 4423–6.
83. Sobotka PA, McMannis J, Fisher RI, Stein DG, Thomas JX Jr. Effects of interleukin 2 on cardiac function in the isolated rat heart. J Clin Invest 1990; 86: 845–50.
84. Vaitkus PT, Grossman D, Fox KR, McEvoy MD, Doherty JU. Complete heart block due to interleukin-2 therapy. Heart 1990; 119: 978–80.
85. Ognibene FP, Rosenberg SA, Lotze M, Skibber J, Parker MM, Shelhamen JH et al. Interleukin-2 administration causes reversible hemodynamic changes and left ventricular dysfunction similar to those seen in septic shock. Chest 1988; 94: 750–4.
86. Sultzer BM. Genetic control of leucocyte responses to endotoxin. Nature 1968; 219: 1253–4.
87. Filkins JP. Monokines and the metabolic pathophysiology of septic shock. Fed Proc 1985; 44: 300–4.
88. Weinberg JR, Wright DJ, Guz A. Interleukin-1 and tumour necrosis factor cause hypotension in the conscious rabbit. Clin Sci 1988; 75: 251–5.
89. Hack CE, De Groot ER, Felt-Bermsa RJF, Nuijens JH, Strack Van Schijndel RJ, Eevenberg-Belmer AJ et al. Increased plasma levels of interleukin-6 in sepsis. Blood 1989; 74: 1704–10.
90. Ikeda U, Ohkawa F, Seino Y, Yamamoto K, Hidaka Y, Kasahara T et al. Serum interleukin 6 levels become elevated in acute myocardial infarction. J Mol Cell Cardiol 1992; 24: 579–84.
91. Hattler BG, Gorcsan J III, Shah N, Oddis CV, Billiar TR, Simmons RL et al. A potential role for nitric oxide (NO) in myocardial stunning. J Card Surg 1994; In press.
92. Finkel MS, Oddis CV, Hattler BG, Simmons RL. Cytokine-mediated myocardial dysfunction. J Immunol Immunopharmacol 1994; In press.
93. Finkel MS, Romeo RC, Oddis CV, Salama G. Inotropic effects of calcium antagonists in the cardiomyopathic Syrian hamster. J Cardiovasc Pharmacol 1992; 19: 546–53.
94. Finkel MS, Shen L, Romeo RC, Oddis CV, Salama G. Radioligand binding and inotropic effects of ryanodine in the cardiomyopathic Syrian hamster. J Cardiovasc Pharmacol 1992; 19: 610–7.
95. Finkel MS, Shen L, Oddis CV, Romeo RC. Verapamil regulation of a defective SR release channel in the cardiomyopathic Syrian hamster. Life Sci 1993; 52: 1109–19.
96. Braunwald E, Rutherford JD. Reversible ischemic left ventricular dysfunction: Evidence for the 'hibernating myocardium'. J Am Coll Cardiol 1986; 8: 1467–70.
97. Capasso JM, Sonnenblick EH, Anversa P. Chronic calcium channel blockade prevents the progression of myocardial contractile and electrical dysfunction in the cardiomyopathic Syrian hamster. Circ Res 1990; 67: 1381–93.
98. Wiedenhold KF, Nilius B. Increased sensitivity of ventricular myocardium in intracellular calcium-overload in Syrian cardiomyopathic hamster. Biomed Biochim Acta 1986; 45: 1333–7.
99. Factor SM, Minase T, Cho S, Dominitz R, Sonnenblick EH. Microvascular spasm in the cardiomyopathic Syrian hamster: A preventable cause of focal myocardial necrosis. Circulation 1982; 66: 342–54.
100. Sonnenblick EH, Fein F, Capasso JM, Factor SM. Microvascular spasm as a cause of cardiomyopathies and the calcium-blocking agent verapamil as potential primary therapy. Am J Cardiol 1985; 55: 179B–184B.

3. Thallium-201 to assess myocardial viability

LYNNE L. JOHNSON

Introduction

This chapter will address the subject of how thallium works as a viability agent both in patients with stable ischemic heart disease and in patients with acute myocardial infarction. There are three groups of patients in whom it is necessary to identify myocardium with contractile dysfunction that is metabolically viable in order to rationally plan management strategies. The first group comprises patients with chronic ischemic heart disease and moderately to severely reduced global left ventricular function. Some patients in this group show improvement in regional and/or global left ventricular wall motion following successful revascularization, while there are others in whom restoration of flow does not improve regional or global wall motion because the heart muscle is predominantly scarred. Operative risk for revascularization in these latter patients is very high and the benefits negligible. They should appropriately be managed medically or undergo orthotopic cardiac transplantation. The second group comprises patients with predominantly single vessel disease and total vessel occlusion with depressed wall motion in the territory of the occluded vessel. The occlusion may have happened suddenly, producing symptomatic acute myocardial infarction, or it may have occurred gradually, without producing symptoms, and found on coronary angiography associated with variable degree of collateral supply to the vascular bed. It is important clinically in these patients as well as the first group to know whether the dyssynergy represents scar from an old silent MI or whether the dyssynergic myocardium is predominantly viable. The third group of patients in whom it is important to identify myocardium with contractile dysfunction that is metabolically viable comprises patients in the early post-myocardial infraction period. Thrombolytic therapy may be initially successful but the infarct vessel may reocclude in the days following the infarction. Alternatively, thrombolytic therapy may never be given and the infarct vessel found to be closed at catheterization sometime during the hospital course. Should 'rescue angioplasty' be performed? Within this group of post-infarction patients there are probably some patients with residual noninfarcted myocardium in the territory of the infarct vessel while there are other patients who have a completed infarction and scar.

The degree of dyssynergy cannot predict viability. Some severely hypokinetic or akinetic segments in the distribution of completely or almost completely

A.S. Iskandrian and E.E. van der Wall (eds): Myocardial viability, 19–37.
© 1994 *Kluwer Academic Publishers.*

occluded coronary arteries can improve function after revascularization [1]. Conversely, a mildly hypokinetic segment resulting from a nontransmural infarction may never become completely normal, even with restoration of flow. Methods to detect myocardial viability were developed years ago, based on the response of a dyssynergic segment either to reduced afterload and increased collateral flow following nitroglycerin administration or based on response to increased inotropic stimulation using post-extrasystolic potentiation [2–4]. These approaches are now finding renewed interest as dobutamine infusion during echocardiographic imaging or perfusion imaging before and after nitroglycerin administration [5–7]. The numbers of patients reported in earlier as well as more recent papers were small. Earlier work suggested that a positive wall motion response to inotropic stimulation was a useful predictor of improvement in wall motion following revascularization but that a negative response did not exclude the possibility of improvement. It is possible that in a heart with globally limited flow, increasing demand through inotropic stimulation will only worsen the flow/demand balance and result in worsening of regional function due to ischemia. These topics are discussed in greater detail elsewhere in this book.

The words 'hibernation' and 'stunning' were coined by astute observers and have become useful descriptive terms implying what may be going on at the cellular level in myocardium that is dysfunctional but not scarred [8, 9]. 'Hibernation' implies that the heart is lying dormant with all metabolic processes down-regulated to meet the simplest primary demands of the cells to just stay alive. 'Stunning' implies that the heart has been hit by an ischemic insult and, following this hit, is lying on the mat, so to speak, waiting for the effects of the blow to wear off before returning to normal function. Subcellular changes that occur in stunned myocardium and which may explain the contractile dysfunction have been described in animal models [10]. There is however, no good animal model for hibernation. It is presumed that as a consequence of severe flow limitation, contractility is reduced as some kind of autoregulation to reduce oxygen demand.

Since the coinage of these two terms, 'hibernation' has been applied to hearts with chronic ischemic disease and depressed left ventricular function while 'stunning' has been applied to hearts that have suffered acute ischemic insults. The application of these two terms may be changing in light of a recently published study in which the investigators carefully measured blood flow, metabolism, and histopathology in a selected group of patients without infarction, and predominantly single vessel disease with total vessel occlusion and collateral dependency of the vascular bed [11]. These investigators found that absolute levels of resting blood flow measured by N-13 ammonia were not reduced in the collateral dependent bed, although flow reserve was markedly reduced. There was a slight increase in rate of exogenous glucose utilization, and there were subcellular structural changes consistent with ischemic insults. Despite the abnormalities in subcellular morphology, the walls improved function following revascularization. The investigators concluded that in these patients with total vessel occlusion and collateral dependent bed, the presence of regional dysfunction is due to repeated episodes of ischemia and therefore an example of stunning rather than hibernation. In light of these data, the term 'stunning' may become more widely applied. It is still possible that in some hearts with severe multivessel disease and globally depressed left ventricular function there is diameter reduction of all major epicardial coronary vessels of such a degree that resting flow is globally reduced and that, as a consequence, function is reduced to restore the balance between supply and demand. Further studies utilizing PET technology are needed to continue to work out the mechanisms underlying depressed regional or global myocardial function in the patient groups described above.

Thallium-201 biokinetics

The biokinetics of thallium have been well worked out by a number of investigators over the past 20 years. Thallium-201 is a cationic element which distributes in the myocardium according to regional blood flow and is taken up into myocytes by an active metabolic process. Because it is a potassium analog, myocardial uptake of thallium is largely dependent on the functioning of the sodium-potassium ATPase pump. That an active metabolic process is necessary for thallium uptake is key to understanding its importance as a viability agent (Table 3.1). Other properties of thallium that aid in its usefulness as a myocardial viability agent include a property common to all diffusible indicators which is increased extraction at low flows. The slow transit time of the tracer through myocardial regions with low flow offer greater opportunity for tracer uptake. The third property of thallium that aids in its usefulness as amyocardial viability agent is redistribution. In the early days of thallium imaging, two doses of tracer were given on two separate days, one at peak stress, the second at rest. It was observed by Pohost *et al.* that fill-in of an ischemic defect occurred if serial imaging was performed following the early stress injection [12]. Further studies showed that redistribution has two components: differential washout and reuptake of thallium from persistent circulating blood levels. The rate of washout of thallium is related to the level of myocardial blood flow, the higher the flow, the faster the washout and the lower the flow, the slower the washout. More rapid washout from normal segments and slower washout from ischemic segments contribute to equalizing counts in the myocardium on delayed images [13]. In addition to differential washout, reuptake of thallium into low flow myocardium from persistent blood levels

Table 3.1. Properties of thallium making it a good viability agent

1. Uptake largely dependent on active metabolic process
2. Increased extraction at low flows
3. Redistribution

also occurs [14]. There is probably a range of thallium blood levels among patients, some maintaining relatively high blood thallium levels, making thallium available for uptake over time into low flow myocardial segments, while other patients have rapid falls in blood thallium levels following initial injections, leaving little or no thallium available for further myocardial uptake. Blood thallium levels may be boosted by thallium reinjection which will be discussed later.

Animal studies have been performed to simulate conditions observed in patients to assess how thallium uptake may relate to myocardial viability in the following situations: coronary occlusion and reflow, myocardial stunning, and low flow state. In an animal model of occlusion and reperfusion, when thallium is given immediately after restoration of flow, thallium uptake occurs in the distribution of hyperemic reflow and underestimates myocardial scar [15, 16]. The thallium defect is smaller in extent than the size of the necrotic segment because thallium is taken up into a rim of perfused but ultimately nonviable myocardium. One would suspect therefore that conclusions cannot be made on the extent of viable/infarcted tissue if thallium is injected immediately after reperfusion.

Moore *et al.* produced myocardial stunning in a canine model by repeated periods of occlusion and reflow [17]. These investigators observed that thallium uptake and washout in the dysfunctional (stunned) myocardial segment was not different from uptake and washout in myocardium with normal wall motion supplied by a stenotic vessel. Based on these results one would conclude that thallium uptake does identify viable myocardium in the clinical setting of stunning. It may be important to mention however that in the recently published study of Vanoverschelde *et al.* in which the investigators used N-13 ammonia as the perfusion tracer, they found that although absolute blood flow in the dysfunctional ('stunned') myocardial segment was normal, that the blood flow to the adjacent normal myocardium was actually higher than normal [11]. Thallium scans give us a picture only of the relative distribution of tracer. If the patients in Vanoverschelde's study had undergone thallium imaging they would probably have shown resting thallium perfusion defects. These defects would however likely show evidence for viability based on redistribution or based on activity levels.

Sinusas and colleagues produced short term 'hibernation' by producing low flow for one hour in a canine model [18]. Despite reduction in flow to 38%, myocardial uptake of thallium was preserved in this low flow non-necrotic model. It is difficult to extrapolate these data to the situation in patients with multivessel disease and globally depressed LV function. Although measurements of absolute myocardial blood flow in man require PET technology, quantitation of thallium uptake and presence of redistribution and/or fill in with reinjection into myocardial segments with low (but observable) thallium uptake on early images have correlated well with viability based on recovery in wall motion following revascularization or by PET metabolic imaging.

Criteria for determining myocardial viability from thallium scans

Homogeneous myocardial uptake of thallium on early images is good evidence that the myocardium imaged is viable. It is possible to imagine a situation in which a diffuse subendocardial infarction has occurred rendering a subendocardial shell of scarred muscle and leaving an epicardial shell of viable muscle. Because the images are not gated and the resolution of the cameras not good enough to resolve across the wall of the left ventricle, such a heart could theoretically appear to have 'normal' thallium uptake. However there would probably be other scan evidence of the subendocardial infarction such as cavitary dilatation. This unlikely situation aside, normal thallium uptake on early scans and the presence of thallium redistribution on delayed scans both indicate myocardial viability.

Although four-hour redistribution thallium imaging is accurate for detecting ischemic heart disease based on the presence of a defect on initial scans and accurate in the majority of cases for diagnosing ischemia based on defect reversibility, it is not accurate for distinguishing between ischemia and scar. Myocardial segments that show redistribution over 4 hours are ischemic and viable, however, a fixed defect on a 4-hour scan does not necessarily mean that the segment is scarred. Several groups of investigators published papers making this observation [19, 20]. Blood *et al.* in the 1970's compared stress and delayed images with stress and second-day rest images, and found that there were significantly fewer defects on the rest images when compared to the redistribution images [21]. Using increased thallium uptake following revascularization as evidence of myocardial viability, several groups of investigators found that from 45% to as high as 83% of irreversible or partially reversible defects on four-hour delayed images showed normal thallium uptake following revascularization [19, 20, 22]. By performing quantitative planar analysis, Gibson *et al.* found that fixed defects with greater than 50% of peak activity for the heart predicted viability as manifest by normalization of thallium uptake following revascularization [22].

It is important to differentiate between the terms 'partially reversible' and 'nonreversible'. The term 'partially reversible' can mean that there is some fill-in at the periphery of the defect, for instance, in the case of an extensive inferior defect which on tomographic images involves the entire inferior, inferoseptal, and inferolateral walls and when at four hours, there is redistribution into the distal and basal defect borders. Some physicians call this type of redistribution 'periinfarction ischemia'. The term 'partial redistribution' is also used when the entire extent of the defect redistributes partially over four hours but does not 'normalize' completely. It would be better to refer to the first situation as both fixed and reversible defects in the affected vascular territory and refer to the second situation as partial redistribution.

There are several different reasons why some ischemic but viable myocardial segments do not redistribute over four hours following the stress injection. Some myocardial segments may be supplied by severely stenotic or occluded vessels without adequate collaterals and, with stress, become so profoundly ischemic that both the severity of the defect and the anatomical limitations to tracer delivery delay redistribution. The other variable operative in determining the rate of redistribution is thallium blood levels which probably vary significantly among patients. Recognizing the limitations of four-hour thallium redistribution to distinguish between viable ischemic myocardium and scar, investigators have pursued two separate approaches to improving the accuracy of thallium imaging to identify myocardial viability.

The first approach is to allow longer time for thallium redistribution to occur by repeating imaging at 18–72 hours after the stress imaging. In this protocol, three sets of images are acquired: early, four-hour delayed, and late (24-hour) imaging. Kiat *et al.* performed tomographic thallium imaging on 21 patients before and after revascularization [23]. Sixty-one percent of defects were nonreversible at four hours and of these nonreversible defects, 61% showed late reversibility. Ninety-five percent of segments showing late reversibility also showed increased thallium uptake after revascularization indicating viability, whereas 37% of the late nonreversible defects were associated with improvement in thallium uptake following revascularization. These findings were further supported in a larger and nonselected population in a study performed by Yang *et al.* [24]. When compared to four-hour delayed imaging, late delayed imaging

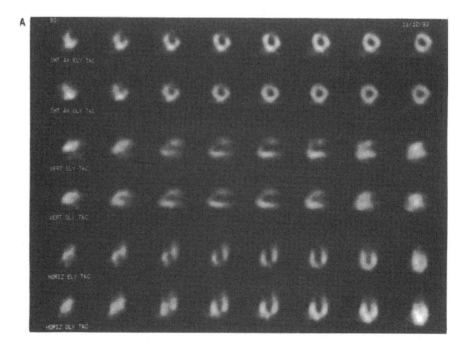

Figure 3.1. Stress, delayed, and reinjection thallium tomographic slices from a patient S/P placement of a stent to the LAD with recurrent chest pain. In each panel the short axis slices are displayed in the top two rows from apex to base (left to right), the vertical long axis slices in the middle two rows from lateral wall to septum, and the horizontal long axis slices in the bottom two

improved the accuracy of thallium imaging to detect myocardial viability, however, there were still a significant number of nonreversible segments at late imaging (37%) which showed post-intervention improvement. In addition, counting statistics can be low at 24 hours, especially in obese patients and in patients with low initial thallium activity in the myocardium.

For the above reasons, a different approach to using thallium to identify myocardial viability was developed by the group at the NIH. This approach is to make more thallium available for myocardial uptake by boosting thallium blood levels by reinjecting a smaller dose of thallium immediately following the four-hour delayed images and performing a third set of images following the reinjection. In the first paper published by this group, 100 patients were studied [25]. There was a wide range of resting left ventricular function in these patients. Left ventricular ejection fraction ranged from 16–69% with a mean of 44% and was reduced below normal in 50 patients. Thirty-three percent of defects were nonreversible at 3 hours and 49% of these showed improved or normal thallium uptake following reinjection. Only 20 of these 100 patients underwent revascularization. Of the 15 segments showing evidence for viability based on increased thallium uptake following reinjection, 13 also showed improvement in regional wall motion following revascularization whereas 8 segments which did not show increased thallium uptake after reinjection did not improve function

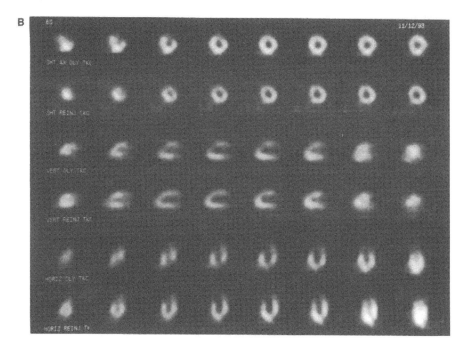

rows from superior to inferior. A) stress and 4-hour redistribution studies are displayed and B) the 4-hour delayed and reinjection studies are displayed. An anteroapical defect is seen on the early studies and shows some redistribution at 4 hours (mid anterior wall). Following reinjection of 1 mCi of thallium the defect is completely resolved.

with revascularization. Other investigators have corroborated the findings of Dilsizian and colleagues supporting the value of thallium reinjection to identify reversible segments [26, 27] (Figure 3.1).

A series of papers were subsequently published examining various alternative protocol options. One option investigated by the NIH group was to eliminate the 3–4 hour redistribution images and reinject thallium at 4 hours and re-image [28]. Using this protocol, the investigators observed apparent 'washout' of thallium following reinjection in a small number of the total stress-induced defects (8%) which, however, represented a fairly large percentage of defects showing 4-hour redistribution (25%). When thallium is injected at rest, myocardial uptake following injection will occur in the distribution of resting myocardial blood flow. In some patients, following thallium reinjection, the higher differential uptake of tracer in the more normally perfused myocardial segments will 'hide' the redistribution observed on the 4-hour delayed images. The conclusion of this study was that there are two imaging options: stress, delayed, reinjection, or stress, reinjection, 24-hour delayed imaging. Time has to be allowed either following the initial injection or following the reinjection for redistribution to occur.

This same group of investigators performed a study to determine whether it is necessary to perform 24-hour imaging after thallium reinjection compared to performing imaging immediately after thallium reinjection [29]. They found that 24-hour imaging following thallium reinjection showed tracer fill-in in only 4 of 35 segments that were irreversible following reinjection and concluded that imaging following reinjection is sufficient to detect myocardial viability. When directly comparing late-delayed (24-hour) imaging to imaging following reinjection, another group of investigators found that significantly more reversible segments are observed when imaging is performed following reinjection of thallium at 24 hours than is found when the 24-hour images alone are compared with the early images [30]. If three sets of images cannot be performed in one day for logistic reasons, the patient may come back on the following day, be reinjected with thallium and re-imaged.

The final protocol option explored is to reinject thallium immediately following the post-exercise study. Two groups have reported results of studies evaluating this protocol and one reported that the approach is not successful while a second group reported that imaging one hour following early thallium reinjection detected more defect reversibility than 3-hour imaging following early thallium reinjection [31, 32]. In this latter study there was no independent measures of myocardial viability and early reinjection was not directly compared to reinjection following 3–4-hour delayed imaging.

Clinically the group of patients in whom differentiating ischemia from scar is most important is the group with multivessel disease and depressed left ventricular function. For this reason, the NIH group went on to address the value of thallium reinjection with quantitation in a group of 16 patients with ischemic heart disease and mean ejection fraction of 27% [33]. These patients underwent treadmill stress and early, 3-hour delayed, and reinjection imaging.

The gold standard for viability in this study was PET metabolic imaging using FDG. The investigators found that following thallium reinjection, thallium activity increased in 47% of defects that were irreversible at 3 hours, but that 59% of defects that were still 'fixed' after thallium reinjection were viable based on FDG uptake. Defects that were fixed following thallium reinjection were divided into subgroups based on severity of count reduction: mild (60–84% peak activity), moderate (50–59% peak activity), severe (< 50% peak activity). Using the quantitative information from the reinjection images, concordance between thallium and PET rose to 88%. Among the irreversible thallium defects with severe count reduction, only 17% showed FDG/blood flow mismatch or an ischemic but viable pattern.

The importance of performing quantitation to identify myocardial viability has been demonstrated by other investigators [1]. When the presence or absence of viability and not presence or absence of ischemia is the clinical question being asked and levels of thallium activity indicate viability or nonviability, then stressing the heart is really not necessary. Ragosta *et al.* performed quantitative analysis on planar scans obtained on 21 patients without recent myocardial infarction with reduced left ventricular ejection fractions, immediately following thallium injection at rest and 3 hours later (rest and redistribution) [34]. The investigators grouped scan patterns into three viability classifications. Normal viability included normal thallium uptake at rest, mild defects on early images which show complete redistribution, and severe defects on early images which show complete redistribution. Mildly reduced viability included mild defects on early images which show partial redistribution, severe defects on early images which show partial redistribution, and mild fixed defects. Severely reduced viability included severe fixed defects. Pre- and post-operative planar thallium scans and gated blood pool scintigrams were performed on each patient. These investigators found that this kind of segment classification into normal, mildly, and severely reduced viability helped predict post revascularization improvement in regional wall motion even in akinetic segments. Whereas the severity of regional wall motion pre-operatively did not predict post-operative improvement in wall motion, viability classification based on quantitative thallium analysis did predict post-operative improvement in regional left ventricular function. Sixty-two percent of severely asynergic segments showing normal viability by thallium improved function after revascularization and 54% of asynergic segments with mild reduction in viability by thallium criteria improved function after revascularization. The greatest improvement in global left ventricular ejection fraction following revascularization occurred in hearts with the greatest number of asynergic viable segments pre-operatively. The predictive value of a pre-operative scan classified as showing evidence for viability for predicting improvement in regional wall motion following revascularization was 73%. These results were confirmed in a similar study by More *et al.* [35].

To summarize the studies described above, myocardial viability can be identified from any one or combination of the following findings; normal

Table 3.2. Criteria for determining myocardial viability from thallium scans

---

1. Normal thallium uptake on early scan
2. Complete thallium redistribution on delayed images
3. Defect fill-in following thallium reinjection
4. Partial redistribution of an initial defect on delayed images if defect cts > 50% peak counts
5. Mild fixed defect with defect cts > 50% peak cts

---

thallium uptake on initial images, complete redistribution of an initial defect on delayed images, partial redistribution of an initial defect on delayed images if the counts in the defect on the delayed images are > 50% of peak activity in the heart, mildly reduced thallium activity (> 50% of peak counts) in a defect that is fixed on four hour imaging, defect fill-in following thallium reinjection. (Table 3.2). It has become the practice in many laboratories that are performing predominantly thallium imaging, to evaluate the early images in the middle of the day and make decisions about whether or not to perform thallium reinjection based on the extent of the defect and the severity of thallium activity reduction in the early defect(s). When information is needed on both ischemia and viability, then the protocol of choice is stress, redistribution, and reinjection. When information is needed on viability only, then rest and redistribution imaging is sufficient. Data available from published studies indicate that a stress, redistribution, reinjection protocol and a rest redistribution protocol are probably equally accurate for detecting myocardial viability. Performing quantitation is important. Most computer systems have either logarithmic or linear color scales with a color change at about 50% of peak activity for the heart. Such a color scale is very useful for localizing as well as assessing the extent of myocardium with reduced thallium activity but with high likelihood for being viable (Figure 3.2).

Assessing myocardial viability in the early post-infarction period

Patients with acute myocardial infarction who undergo early, successful reperfusion of the infarct related artery either by thrombolytic therapy or by balloon angioplasty should be left with only a small non-Q wave infarction and no myocardium at further ischemic risk. There are, however, a variety of factors that may change this picture and leave a patient with myocardium at risk and they include the following: reocclusion of the infarct-related vessel, residual tight stenosis in the infarct-related artery following successful thrombolysis, or multivessel disease with myocardium at risk remote from the infarct territory. Although combining perfusion imaging with some kind of stress would probably increase the sensitivity for detecting myocardium at ischemic risk, it would be optimal to risk-stratify patients very early in their post-infarction course, perhaps at the time of discharge from the CCU when plans for either routine noninvasive predischarge risk-stratification or coronary angiography

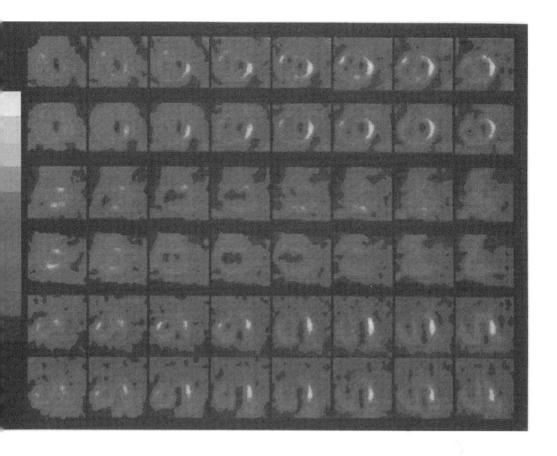

Figure 3.2. Display of tomographic images from a patient with multivessel CAD and severe LV dysfunction and pulmonary hypertension. The display format and orientation are the same as in Figure 3.1. The 10-color scale assigns to the highest counts shades of white through yellow, gold, red, purple and black represents 0 counts. Myocardial segments with dark orange and hotter colors have counts > 50% peak activity for the heart. The highest counts in this patient's heart are in the lateral wall of the LV. The entire LAD territory (anterior wall, septum) has severely reduced counts corresponding to extensive scar in this vascular territory. The inferior wall has only moderately reduced counts, just above 50% of the lateral wall, therefore fulfilling the criteria for viability. The RV is very prominent.

can be planned. Although pharmacologic stress perfusion imaging with thallium for risk-stratification post-infarction has been performed and reported in a fairly large patient population [36, 37], it has not been performed as early as 2 days post-infarction when complications related to pharmacologic vasodilation may be more frequent and less readily reversible.

An alternative approach is to perform rest thallium imaging in the early post-infarction period and assess viability based on quantitative techniques and/or presence of redistribution on delayed images. Differentiating between hypoperfused (ischemic) and stunned myocardium in this setting may be difficult, and distinguishing between these two pathologic conditions may have more clinical importance than in patients which ischemic heart disease and no recent myocardial infarction. As reported earlier in this chapter, animal studies of acutely stunned myocardium have shown normal thallium uptake and patient studies of chronically stunned myocardium have also shown normal values for myocardial blood flow measured by N-13 ammonia. It is possible however, that blood flow to myocardium remote from the infarct zone may be higher than normal, making the stunned segment with normal, absolute blood flow appear as a defect. A defect appearing on a resting scan performed in the early post-infarction period could therefore represent one of several pathological conditions: transmural scar, nontransmural scar, viable hypoperfused myocardium, viable stunned myocardium (Table 3.3). The simultaneous imaging of an infarct avid tracer which demarcates regions of necrosis may help identify the scarred segments.

Antimyosin is an Fab fragment of a murine monoclonal antibody produced by hybridoma technology and directed against human heavy chain cardiac myosin. In a series of *in vitro* studies, Khaw and colleagues demonstrated that antimyosin uptake is highly specific for myocyte necrosis [38, 39]. For antimyosin to gain access and bind with myosin, the cell membrane must become disrupted, a change that signals irreversible myocyte injury. Antimyosin is bound via the chelator DTPA to indium-111, a gamma emitter with a 67-hour half-life and two photopeaks, at 167 and 247 keV. Because the antibody fragment is a fairly large protein molecule, it clears from the blood pool relatively slowly. The T1/2 for the major component of the blood clearance curve in man is 6–12 hours [40]. In addition to necrotic myocardium, tracer uptake occurs in the liver and kidneys (route of excretion). Indium-111 and thallium-201 are well suited for simultaneous imaging because the half-lives of the two tracers are almost the same and, therefore' the administered doses are equivalent.

In a dog infarct model, both indium-111 antimyosin and thallium were injected and *in vivo* tomographic imaging performed [41]. Half of the animals underwent a 2-hour balloon occlusion followed by reflow and the other half underwent a 6-hour balloon occlusion (approximating a 'no reflow state') followed by balloon deflation. Indium-111 antimyosin was injected soon after balloon deflation and 24 hours later (to allow for blood pool clearance), thallium was injected and the animals underwent simultaneous dual isotope tomographic imaging using the high photopeak of indium-111 and the 70 keV photopeak of thallium. Because the lower photopeak of indium-111 is close to

Table 3.3. Pathological conditions producing thallium defects early post-mi

---

1. Transmural scar
2. Nontransmural scar
3. Viable hypoperfused myocardium
4. Viable stunned myocardium

---

the high photopeak of thallium and although the percentage of the total thallium counts in this photopeak is small, the relative percentage of thallium to indium counts is high and therefore the lower photopeak of indium-111 was not used. The two simultaneously acquired tomographic slices were displayed side by side on a computer screen and regions of thallium uptake correlated with regions of antimyosin uptake. In animals with 6-hour occlusion, the infarctions were predominantly transmural, the thallium activity very low or absent and the antimyosin uptake although present was faint probably due to microvascular occlusion limiting antimyosin delivery. Regions of antimyosin uptake fit into the thallium defects like pieces of a puzzle. The 2-hour occlusion infarcts were nontransmural. The thallium defects showed mild to moderate count reduction, on histopathology the infarctions were nontransmural, and on imaging there was some degree of overlap of the two tracers in the infarct zone. Antimyosin uptake was more intense in this model than in the 6-hour occlusion model probably due to unimpeded delivery of the radiotracer into the infarct zone. The results of these experimental studies documented that simultaneous tomographic imaging of these two tracers can be performed and the results offer useful information on necrosis and viability. Consequently, 87 patients admitted to the coronary care unit at Columbia Presbyterian Medical Center with acute ischemic syndromes were injected with indium-111 antimyosin and thallium [42]. The study population comprised 61 patients with acute Q-wave infarctions, 17 with non-Q-wave infarctions, 3 with nonlocalizable infarctions due to intraventricular conduction defects, and 6 with unstable angina. Because of the nature of the referral population, an inner city hospital with poor and/or elderly patients who tend to arrive at the hospital late in the course of their infarctions, only 10/87 qualified for thrombolytic therapy. Patients were injected with 2.0 mCi of indium-111 antimyosin at the bedside as soon as the diagnosis of myocardial infarction was confirmed by enzyme or ECG changes. Forty-eight hours later the patients were brought to the nuclear cardiology laboratory and injected with 2.2 mCi of thallium and underwent simultaneous dual isotope tomographic acquisition using a single detector camera acquiring 32 images over 180° at 60 sec per step for a total imaging time of 35 minutes. This acquisition time which is longer than for a standard thallium acquisition is necessary to get good counting statistics for both radiotracers using a medium energy collimator.

The thallium tomograms were reconstructed first and the same oblique angles of rotation were used to reconstruct the indium antimyosin tomograms. Performing oblique tomographic reconstruction on the indium antimyosin raw data alone, without the aid of the thallium data, in most cases would be impossible because the axes of the heart cannot be identified from infarct tracer uptake alone. The simultaneously acquired tomographic slices were displayed on a computer screen side by side and the uptake of thallium and indium antimyosin marked on worksheets. Three patterns of uptake of the two tracers were observed and classified as matches, mismatches, or overlap. In a matching pattern, the location and extent of the indium antimyosin uptake corresponded

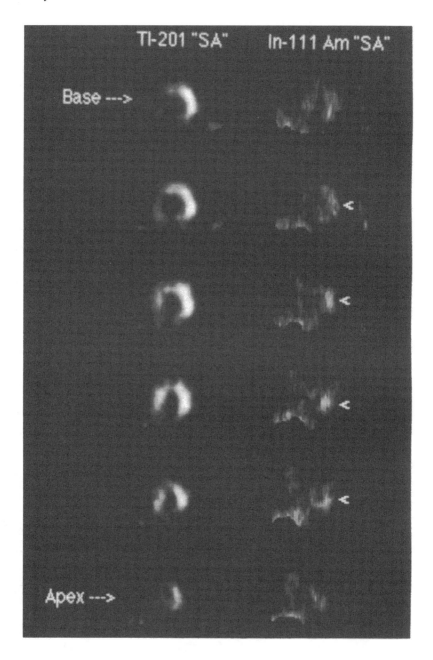

Figure 3.3. Short axis tomographic slices of simultaneous dual isotope (thallium-201 and indium-111 antimyosin antibody) tomographic acquisitions showing multiple patterns of relative uptake of the two tracers. The patient had a history of a remote inferior infarction, was admitted with an acute non-Q lateral wall infarction. The antimyosin uptake (arrows) is in the lateral wall of the LV where thallium uptake is greatest (overlap). There is an inferior thallium defect without antimyosin uptake (mismatch) in the territory of the old inferior infarction. In addition, there is a mild anteroseptal and

to the location and extent of the thallium defect. Most of these patients had sustained acute Q-wave infarctions. In a mismatching pattern, the extent of the thallium defect was greater than the extent of the indium antimyosin uptake. Some patients showing this pattern had histories of remote myocardial infarctions. In other patients, the hypoperfused myocardial segments were probably due to one of two mechanisms, either hypoperfusion due to a severe residual coronary artery stenosis and poor collaterals limiting delivery of thallium, stunning where flow is close to normal but less than flow to remote noninfarcted segments, failure of antimyosin to reach the infarct territory due to microvascular damage (no reflow) within the infarct territory, or total occlusion of the infarct related artery and absent collaterals (false-negative antimyosin scan). The third pattern observed was overlap of the two tracers in the same myocardial walls. The explanation for this finding is simpler. It most likely represents nontransmural necrosis. To support this explanation, this pattern was most frequently seen in patients who had sustained non-Q-wave infarctions. Many patients had more than one scan pattern in their hearts. For instance, a match or overlap was seen in one vascular territory and mismatch in another (Figure 3.3).

In an attempt to use these scan patterns to risk-stratify patients early in their post-infarction hospital course, both the mismatch pattern and the overlap pattern were designated to potentially indicate myocardium at further ischemic risk and the matching pattern designated to indicate a completed transmural infarction without myocardium at further ischemic risk. All patients were followed for 6 weeks and the ischemic endpoints were defined as death, infarct extension, recurrent infarction, recurrent angina leading to catheterization, ischemia detected on the predischarge low level or 6-week, symptom-limited treadmill stress test. Using these clinical endpoints, 39 of 87 patients had further ischemia which included the following: death in 3, infarct extension or recurrence in 4, chest pain leading to catheterization in 22, ischemic pulmonary edema in 2, and positive treadmill ECG stress tests in 8. Thirty-eight of the 39 patients with further ischemia had either mismatch and/or overlap on their scans leading to a very high sensitivity of this test to identify patients with further ischemic risk.

All 27 patients with only a matching pattern on scans were event-free. However, there were another 21 patients with mismatch and/or overlap who did not show further evidence for ischemia up to 6 weeks, giving the test a low specificity. There are a variety of factors contributing to these 'false-positive' scan patterns. Some patients had false-negative antimyosin scans. Some had an unmatched thallium defect in the distribution of a remote myocardial infarction. Some, however, may have had myocardium at further risk but did not become symptomatic. For instance, there were 6 patients with anterior infarctions and a partially unmatched thallium defect in the infarct territory. All

---

apical thallium defect which redistributed at 4 hours. The results of these scans were not used to guide patient management and the patient went on to have a recurrent ischemic event.

of these patients underwent coronary angiography which documented complete occlusion of the infarct vessel. One could hypothesize that there was residual viable myocardium in the infarct territory and that rescue angioplasty would help preserve this function. Unfortunately, quantitative analysis was not performed on these studies. It would have been very interesting to quantitate the thallium activity in the unmatched thallium defects. When combined with the antimyosin uptake and localization, it may help to differentiate between stunning and ischemia.

Quantitative planar thallium imaging was performed by Sabia *et al.* in patients with totally occluded infarct related arteries following acute myocardial infarction [43]. These investigators performed quantitative planar rest and redistribution thallium imaging and regional wall motion analysis in 57 patients prior to and following attempts to open the vessels. Interestingly, from their data only 11 of 57 patients had mean thallium activity in the thallium defects below 50% of peak activity, which would suggest that the majority still had viable myocardium in the infarct bed. All patients with successful angioplasties showed both improvement in wall motion and increases in thallium activity in the infarct beds, while those with unsuccessful angioplasty did not. Presence or absence of thallium redistribution did not help identify patients who would improve following revascularization.

Fifty-seven of the 87 patients in the dual isotope study also underwent thallium redistribution imaging following the initial set of rest tomograms. Although these 57 patients represented the full spectrum of patients recruited and were not a select group with total occlusion of the infarct related artery, nevertheless, the value of thallium redistribution when compared to the initial dual isotope scans was much less sensitive and only slightly more specific. Although thallium redistribution means viability, lack of thallium redistribution, post-myocardial infarction does not mean nonviability. In fact, reverse thallium redistribution is not infrequently seen in these patients. In reverse redistribution, the thallium defect intensifies between the early and delayed images. The mechanism for this observation is presumed to be due to the fact that thallium is taken up into both normal noninfarcted myocardium and into the epicardial layer in nontransmural infarctions. Over 3 to 4 hours following this initial tracer distribution, there is washout which occurs at normal rates both from the normal noninfarcted tissue and from noninfarcted epicardial component of the nontransmural infarction. Because of equal rates of washout from nonequal masses of myocardium, the infarct zone appears to lose more counts over time compared to the normal zone. Based on published studies to date, most information relating to myocardial viability in patients who have sustained recent myocardial infarctions can be obtained by either combining imaging of a necrosis avid imaging agent with a perfusion tracer and/or performing quantitation on the rest images.

References

1. Beller GA, Ragosta M, Watson DD, Gimple LW. Myocardial thallium-201 scintigraphy for assessment of viability in patients with severe left ventricular dysfunction. Am J Cardiol 1992; 70: 18E–22E.
2. Bodenheimer MM, Banka VS, Hermann GA, Trout RG, Pasdar H, Helfant RH. Reversible asynergy. Histopathologic and electrographic correlations in patients with coronary artery disease. Circulation 1976; 53: 792–6.
3. Dyke SH, Cohn PF, Gorlin R, Sonnenblick EH. Detection of residual myocardial function in coronary artery disease using post-extra systolic potentiation. Circulation 1974; 50: 694–9.
4. Helfant RH, Pine R, Meister SG, Feldman MS, Trout RG, Banka VS. Nitroglycerin to unmask reversible asynergy. Correlation with post coronary bypass ventriculography. Circulation 1974; 50: 108–13.
5. Charney R, Schwinger ME, Cohen MV, Menegus M, Spindola-Franco H, Greensberg MA. Dobutamine echocardiography predicts recovery of hibernating myocardium following coronary revascularization [abstract]. J Am Coll Cardiol 1992; 19 (Suppl A): 176A.
6. Medrano R, Mahmarian JJ, Verani MS. Nitroglycerin before reinjection of thallium-201 enhances detection of reversible hypoperfusion via collateral blood flow: A randomized, double blind, parallel, placebo-controlled trial [abstract]. J Am Coll Cardiol 1993; 21 (Suppl A): 221A.
7. Galli M, Marcassa C, Silva P, Zoccarato O, Campini R. Improvement of resting 99 m Tc-sestamibi myocardial uptake by acute nitroglycerin administration [abstract]. J Am Coll Cardiol 1993; 21 (Suppl A): 221A.
8. Braunwald E, Kloner RA. The stunned myocardium: Prolonged, postischemic ventricular dysfunction. Circulation 1982; 66: 1146–9.
9. Braunwald E, Rutherford JD. Reversible ischemic left ventricular dysfunction: Evidence for the 'hibernating myocardium'. J Am Coll Cardiol 1986; 8: 1467–70.
10. Kusuoka H, Porterfield JK, Weisman HF, Weisfeldt ML, Marban E. Pathophysiology and pathogenesis of stunned myocardium. Depressed Ca^{2+} activation of contraction as a consequence of reperfusion-induced cellular calcium overload in ferre hearts. J Clin Invest 1987; 79: 950–61.
11. Vanoverschelde JL, Wijns W, Depré C, Essamri B, Heyndrickx GR, Borgers M et al. Mechanisms of chronic regional postischemic dysfunction in human. New insights from the study of noninfarcted collateral-dependent myocardium. Circulation 1993; 87: 1513–23.
12. Pohost GM, Zir LM, Moore RH, McKusick KA, Guiney TE, Beller GA. Differentiation of transiently ischemic from infarcted myocardium by serial imaging after a single dose of thallium-201. Circulation 1977; 55: 294–302.
13. Okada RD, Pohost GM. Effect of decreased blood flow and ischemia on myocardial thallium clearance. J Am Coll Cardiol 1984; 3: 744–50.
14. Budinger TF, Pohost GM, Bischoff P. Thallium 201 integral concentration over 2 hours explains persistent defects in patients with no evidence of MI by ECG [abstract]. Circulation 1987; 76 (4 Suppl IV): IV64.
15. Forman R, Kirk ES. Thallium-201 accumulation during reperfusion of ischemic myocardium: Dependence on regional blood flow rather than viability. Am J Cardiol 1984; 54: 659–63.
16. Granato JE, Watson DD, Flanagan TL, Gascho JA, Beller GA. Myocardial thallium-201 kinetics during coronary occlusion and reperfusion: Influence of method of reflow and timing of thallium-201 administration. Circulation 1986; 73: 150–60.
17. Moore CA, Cannon J, Watson DD, Kaul S, Beller GA. Thallium 201 kinetics in stunned myocardium characterized by severe postischemic systolic dysfunction. Circulation 1990; 81: 1622–32.
18. Sinusas AJ, Watson DD, Cannon JM Jr, Beller GA. Effect of ischemia and postischemic dysfunction on myocardial uptake of technetium-99m-labeled methoxyisobutyl isonitrile and thallium-201. J Am Coll Cardiol 1989; 14: 1758–93.

19. Liu P, Kiess MC, Okada RD, Block PC, Strauss HW, Pohost GM *et al.* The persistent defect on exercise thallium imaging and its fate after myocardial revascularization: Does is represent scar or ischemia? Am Heart J 1985; 110: 996–1001.
20. Cloninger KG, DePuey EG, Garcia EV, Roubin GS, Robbins WL, Nody A *et al.* Incomplete redistribution in delayed thallium-201 single photon emission computed tomographic (SPECT) images: An overestimation of myocardial scarring. J Am Coll Cardiol 1988; 12: 955–63.
21. Blood DK, McCarthy DM, Sciacca RR, Cannon PJ. Comparison of single-dose and double-dose thallium-201 myocardial perfusion scintigraphy for the detection of coronary artery disease and prior myocardial infarction. Circulation 1978; 58: 777–88.
22. Gibson RS, Watson DD, Taylor GJ, Crosby IK, Wellons HL, Holt ND *et al.* Prospective assessment of regional myocardial perfusion before and after coronary revascularization surgery by quantitative thallium-201 scintigraphy. J Am Coll Cardiol 1983; 1: 804–15.
23. Kiat H, Berman DS, Maddahi J, De Yang LD, Van Train K, Rozanski A *et al.* Late reversibility of tomographic myocardial thallium-201 defects: An accurate marker of myocardial viability. J Am Coll Cardiol 1988; 12: 1456–63.
24. Yang LD, Berman DS, Kiat H, Ressen KJ, Friedman JD, Rozanski A *et al.* The frequency of late reversibility in SPECT thallium-201 stress redistribution studies. J Am Coll Cardiol 1989; 15: 334–40.
25. Dilsizian V, Rocco TP, Freedman NM, Leon MB, Bonow RO. Enhanced detection of ischemic but viable myocardium by the reinjection of thallium after stress-redistribution imaging. N Engl J Med 1990; 323: 141–6.
26. Ohtani H, Tamaki N, Yonekura Y, Mohiuddin IH, Hirata K, Ban T *et al.* Value of thallium-201 reinjection after delayed SPECT imaging for predicting reversible ischemia after coronary artery bypass grafting. Am J Cardiol 1990; 66: 394–9.
27. Tamaki N, Ohtani H, Yonekura Y, Nohara R, Kambara H, Kawai C *et al.* Significance of fill-in after thallium-201 reinjection following delayed imaging: comparison with regional wall motion and angiographic findings. J Nucl Med 1990; 31: 1617–23.
28. Dilsizian V, Bonow RO. Differential uptake and apparent ^{201}Tl washout after thallium reinjection. Options regarding early redistribution imaging before reinjection or late redistribution imaging after reinjection. Circulation 1992; 85: 1032–8.
29. Dilsizian V, Smeltzer WR, Freedman NM, Dextras R, Bonow RO. Thallium reinjection after stress-redistribution imaging. Does 24-hour delayed imaging after reinjection enhance detection or viable myocardium? Circulation 1991; 83: 1247–55.
30. Kayden DS, Sigal S, Souger R, Mattera J, Zaret BL, Wackers FJ. Thallium-201 for assessment of myocardial viability: Quantitative comparison of 24-hour redistribution imaging with imaging after reinjection at rest. J Am Coll Cardiol 1991; 18: 1480–6.
31. Kiat H, Friedman JD, Wang FP, Van Train KF, Maddahi J, Takemoto K *et al.* Frequency of late reversibility in stress-redistribution thallium-201 SPECT using an early reinjection protocol. Am Heart J 1991; 122: 613–9.
32. van Eck-Smit BL, van der Wall EE, Kuijper AF, Zwinderman AH, Pauwels EK. Immediate thallium-201 reinjection following stress imaging: A time saving approach for detection of myocardial viability. J Nucl Med 1993; 34: 737–43.
33. Bonow RO, Dilsizian V, Cuocolo A, Bacharach SL. Identification of viable myocardium in patients with chronic coronary artery disease and left ventricular dysfunction. Comparison of thallium scintigraphy with reinjection and PET imaging with ^{18}F-Fluorodeoxyglucose. Circulation 1991; 83: 26–37.
34. Ragosta M, Beller GA, Watson DD, Kaul S, Gimple LW. Quantitative planar rest redistribution ^{201}Tl imaging in detection of myocardial viability and prediction of improvement in left ventricular function after coronary bypass surgery in patients with severely depressed left ventricular function. Circulation 1993; 87: 1630–41.
35. Mori T, Minamiji K, Kurogane H, Ogawa K, Yoshida Y. Rest-injected thallium-201 imaging for assessing viability of severe asynergic regions. J Nucl Med 1991; 32: 1718–24.

36. Brown KA, O'Meara J, Chambers CE, Plante DA. Ability of dipyridamole-thallium-201 imaging one to four days after acute myocardial infarction to predict in-hospital and late recurrent myocardial ischemic events. Am J Cardiol 1990; 65: 160–7.
37. Mahmarian JJ, Pratt CM, Nishimura S, Abreu A, Verani MS. Quantitative adenosine 201Tl single-photon emission computed tomography for the early assessment of patients surviving acute myocardial infarction. Circulation 1993; 87: 1197–210.
38. Khaw BA, Fallon JT, Beller GA, Haber E. Specificity of localization of myosin-specific antibody fragments in experimental myocardial infarction. Histologic, histochemical, autoradiographic and scintigraphic studies. Circulation 1979; 60: 1527–31.
39. Khaw BA, Scott J, Fallon JT, Cahill SL, Haber E, Homcy C. Myocardial injury: Quantitation by cell shortening initiated with antimyosin fluorescent spheres. Science 1982; 217: 1050–3.
40. Khaw BA, Yasuda T, Gold HK, Leinbach RC, Johns JA, Kanke M et al. Acute myocardial infarct imaging with indium-111-labeled monoclonal antimyosin Fab. J Nucl Med 1987; 28: 1671–8.
41. Johnson LL, Lerrick KS, Coromilas J, Seldin DW, Esser PD, Zimmerman JM et al. Measurement of infarct size and percentage myocardium infarcted in a dog preparation with single photon-emission computed tomography, thallium-201, and indium 111-monoclonal antimyosin Fab. Circulation 1987; 76: 181–90.
42. Johnson LL, Seldin DW, Keller AM, Wall RM, Bhatia K, Bingham CO 3d et al. Dual isotope thallium and indium antimyosin SPECT imaging to identify acute infarct patients at further ischemic risk. Circulation 1990; 81: 37–45.
43. Sabia PJ, Powers ER, Ragosta M, Smith WH, Watson DD, Kaul S. Role of quantitative planar thallium-201 imaging for determining viability in patients with acute myocardial infarction and a totally occluded infarct-related artery. J Nucl Med 1993; 34: 728–36.

4. The role of technetium-99m Sestamibi in the evaluation of myocardial viability

PIERRE RIGO, THERÈSE BENOIT & SIMON BRAAT

Introduction

The role of technetium-99m (Tc-99m) Sestamibi in the evaluation of myocardial viability has been the subject of some debate [1–3]. Whereas many experimental findings have documented features suggesting the value of Tc-99m Sestamibi in this respect, several clinical reports have shown discordant results or have indicated an apparent superiority of thallium-201. It seems, therefore, important to analyse the value of Tc-99m Sestamibi, taking into account recent clinical and experimental results, as well as the clinical problem.

Defining the clinical problem is the first priority [4,5]. This is especially necessary as the term viability is misleading. Indeed, normal myocardium is by definition viable but we are not really interested in defining normal myocardium. What we are looking for is 'jeopardized' myocardium, that is, dysfunctioning myocardium capable of recovering normal function upon restoration of normal perfusion. The key word in this definition is function. Regions with normal or even slightly abnormal but retained function are viable by definition [6]. Only regions with severely altered or absent residual function need to be explored. Therefore, we believe that the term 'viability' is not optimal and that it should be replaced by 'reversible chronic dysfunction' or 'jeopardized myocardium'.

Differential diagnosis

Differential diagnosis of jeopardized myocardium includes myocardial ischemia, stunning, hibernating myocardium and incomplete infarction. Myocardial ischemia is first under consideration, as it is the most frequent condition leading to transient reversible myocardial dysfunction. Acute, exercise-induced ischemia is clinically easily recognized but unstable angina is definitively part of the differential diagnosis since ischemia is recurrent and silent episodes of ischemia are frequent, and because ischemic dysfunction and/or stunning may persist after the acute ischemic episodes [7].

Stunned myocardium is a condition characterized by persistent dysfunction after reperfusion, following a prolonged episode of ischemia [8,9]. Recovery of function, although delayed for several hours or days, is the rule in stunning. Hibernating myocardium is a chronic condition resulting from reduced flow

A.S. Iskandrian and E.E. van der Wall (eds): Myocardial viability, 39–52.
© 1994 *Kluwer Academic Publishers.*

with concomitant myocardial dysfunction [10]. Myocardial ischemia is probably not part of this condition as myocardial energy requirements are markedly reduced by the reduced rate of contraction; a chronic equilibrium between oxygen and substrate supply and demand that can be maintained. Other theories, however, see hibernating myocardium as the consequence of recurrent ischemic episodes with intercurrent stunning. Whatever its cause, hibernating myocardium appears to be associated with the development of a particular histological picture of cell dedifferentiation with loss of contractile fibers and accumulation of glycogen [11]. Recovery from hibernating myocardium is possible but is frequently delayed and related to the severity and duration of hibernation. Clinical data documenting requirements for reversibility and time course of reversibility in different degrees and extensions of hibernating myocardium are lacking.

Finally, incomplete myocardial infarction must be considered. In the past, incomplete myocardial infarction was equated with nontransmural myocardial infarction or non-Q wave infarct, a somewhat vague yet distinct entity [12]. Nowadays, with the advent of fibrinolysis, classical nontransmural myocardial infarction is rarely encountered. However, fibrinolysis often results in incomplete myocardial infarction probably with a more heterogeneous mixture of salvaged and necrotic myocardium. These regions may appear on scintigrams as regions of fixed, reduced uptake, which reflect an open artery with diminished flow supplying a reduced mass of myocardium. The evolution of function in such regions is difficult to predict as it depends on the size of the infarct and the scarring process. Slow improvement of function is possible, however, as the scar may diminish the size of the infarct over time.

Tools

Several tools are available to detect and identify jeopardized myocardium or reversible chronic dysfunctioning myocardium. As detailed elsewhere in this book, demonstration of retained myocardial metabolic activity is evidence for retained viability and has been used to predict recovery [13]. On the other hand, irreversible scar tissue has minimal residual metabolic activity of all substrates, whether fatty acids, acetate, glucose, ketone bodies, amino acids or oxygen. Ischemic or jeopardized myocardium undergoes metabolic impairment in a progressive manner. First, as oxygen supply diminishes, aerobic metabolism of substrates such as fatty acids, acetate or ketone bodies is affected. Glucose utilization persists longer as glucose can be used both in aerobic and anaerobic fashions. Glucose or fluorine-18 deoxyglucose (FDG) uptake is therefore increased in relation to flow in patients with myocardial ischemia or hibernating myocardium [14]. (Flow is also affected in ischemic or jeopardized myocardium.) Both experimental and clinical studies have shown progressive alteration of flow to correspond with progressive loss of viability and diminished potential for recovery. In fact, some studies have shown that the degree of quantitative flow impairment, as measured by positron emission tomography (PET), was the best parameter to indicate potential for functional recovery in patients with myocardial infarction or ischemia [15–17].

Tracers indicative of membrane integrity such as cations (rubidium-82, potassium-38, and thallium-201) have provided useful indication of myocardial viability [18]. Extraction of cations in myocardial cells is inversely related to flow and, therefore, highest at low and even very low flow. This remains the case in acutely ischemic cells, but these cells cannot retain the tracer thereafter and its release is accelerated. The rate of rubidium-82 and potassium-38 release has been used to indicate nonviable myocardium [18,19].

Potential position of Tc-99m Sestamibi

Based on the previous considerations, the role of Tc-99m Sestamibi as a tracer of viability should be considered from three different points of view regarding its ability to indicate membrane integrity, regional myocardial blood flow and regional ventricular function. In contrast to thallium-201, the volume of distribution of the tracer (especially after redistribution) does not appear to be a valuable parameter.

Tc-99m Sestamibi as a tracer of membrane integrity
Experimental studies have indicated the value of Tc-99m Sestamibi as a tracer of membrane integrity. Initially, myocellular uptake rates of Tc-99m Sestamibi reflect mean plasma membrane potential rather than Na, K-ATPase, as with thallium-201. Once in the cytosol, Tc-99m Sestamibi is further concentrated into the mitochondria [20].

Chick embryo heart cells concentrate Tc-99m Sestamibi 30 to 50 times the extracellular concentration in the steady state. Depolarization of the plasma membrane by changes in the extracellular potassium content reduces the Tc-99m Sestamibi accumulation by a factor of 6. Poisoning or inhibition of the mitochondria (for instance by valinomycin) will abolish accumulation and result in an uptake ratio of 1 [20].

In intact heart cells, the final net accumulation of Tc-99m Sestamibi is approximately 5 times higher than that of thallium-201 (when normalized to equal extracellular concentration). This difference probably reflects the lack of thallium-201 accumulation in the mitochondria. As shown by Piwnica-Worms *et al.* [21], severe myocellular injury completely depletes Tc-99m Sestamibi cell content, while thallium-201 uptake persists around 40% of reference value. Moderate injury already depresses thallium-201 uptake while Tc-99m Sestamibi uptake is transiently enhanced, reflecting hyperpolarization of the cell. Based on these results, in a non-flow dependent preparation Tc-99m Sestamibi can better distinguish reversible from irreversible injuries than thallium-201.

Tc-99m Sestamibi as a tracer of myocardial blood flow

As discussed earlier, evaluation of myocardial blood flow is another approach to discriminate between viable and nonviable regions. The use of Tc-99m Sestamibi as a tracer of myocardial blood flow relies on the Sapirstein principle [22]. Like potassium and thallium-201, Tc-99m Sestamibi has incomplete first pass extraction and the extraction fraction varies with flow [23–27]. It increases at a low flow rate and diminishes at a high flow rate. Compared to thallium-201, Tc-99m Sestamibi has lower peak extraction but similar net extraction, as Tc-99m Sestamibi is subsequently released much slower than thallium-201. Based on Marshall's data [27], Tc-99m Sestamibi net extraction becomes higher than that of thallium-201 after 40 minutes under low flow and 20 minutes under high flow conditions. The ratio of net extraction at high flow versus net extraction at low flow, a potential indication of the ability to visualize flow disparity in myocardial ischemia, decreases faster for thallium-201 than for Tc-99m Sestamibi and the crossover point is reached approximately 20 minutes after injection.

Several studies in the experimental animal have validated the ability of Tc-99m Sestamibi to indicate regional myocardial blood flow [24,26,28]. As with other tracers, the relationship between tracer uptake and flow deteriorates at high flow. But a good correlation between uptake and flow has been observed up to 300 ml/min/100 g with Tc-99m Sestamibi [29]. In studies performed in the setting of an experimental myocardial infarction, however (after coronary occlusion of 3 hours or more followed by reperfusion), that correlation is not maintained in the infarcted tissue (TTC negative tissue) [28,30]. This is in contrast with thallium-201. Indeed, several authors have demonstrated a persistent correlation between thallium-201 uptake and blood flow in the reperfused infarct situation [31]. This correlation is also noted in the TTC negative samples. Therefore, in this setting, thallium-201 appears to follow myocardial blood flow more closely than Tc-99m Sestamibi even though the latter should be a better indicator of myocardial viability.

In studies performed under conditions of low flow and systolic dysfunction, Sinusas *et al.* [32] have compared the uptake of thallium-201 and Tc-99m Sestamibi after 40 minutes of partial occlusion of the left anterior descending coronary artery (LAD), and during reperfusion after 15 minutes of complete occlusion of the LAD. Thallium-201 and Tc-99m Sestamibi activity in the ischemic zone were comparable and proportional to flow. There was a good linear correlation among the endocardial segments between flow and the uptake of thallium-201 ($r = 0.78$) and of Tc-99m Sestamibi ($r = 0.85$). During reperfusion, central ischemic endocardial flow (59 ± 14%) was again comparable to thallium-201 (70 ± 10%) and Tc-99m Sestamibi (74 ± 12%) activity, indicating comparable uptake of both tracers under conditions of low coronary flow and dysfunction.

Using a similar model, the same group more recently reported data on thallium-201 redistribution [33]. In 16 open- chest dogs, the LAD was ligated, leading to a 50% mean flow reduction and a decreased left ventricular thickening from 25.6 +/± 1.7% to ±1.3 ± 2.5%. After 30 minutes of low flow, 1.0 mCi of thallium-201 and microspheres were injected and initial thallium-201 images obtained. After 2 hours, redistribution images were taken and subsequently 10 mCi of Tc-99m Sestamibi and microspheres were injected. LAD/LCX count ratios for both tracers and flow were calculated by well counting after sacrifice. Defect magnitudes of thallium-201 and Tc-99m Sestamibi were determined by quantitative imaging analysis of LAD/LCX count ratios. The flow ratios of LAD/LCX were similar during thallium-201 (0.56 ± 0.04) and Tc-99m Sestamibi (0.58 ± 0.06) injections, however, the activity at redistribution of thallium-201 was significantly higher, indicating increased thallium-201 uptake (0.83 ± 0.03 versus 0.64 ± 0.05). Similarly, the delayed thallium-201 image ratio at redistribution showed higher ischemic over normal count ratio (0.73 ± 0.02) than observed for Tc-99m Sestamibi (0.65 ± 0.02), whereas thallium-201 and Tc-99m Sestamibi magnitude were identical on the initial rest scans. Thus, in this model of sustained low flow and profound systolic dysfunction, thallium-201 redistribution appears to highlight viability while Tc-99m Sestamibi remains a tracer of myocardial blood flow. Both tracers, however, show substantial uptake in severely asynergic myocardium. Also, it should be pointed out that the *in vitro* activity ratio is not completely translated into the image count ratio probably as the result of attenuation and scatter affecting thallium-201 more severely than Tc-99m Sestamibi.

Evaluation of regional myocardial function using Tc-99m Sestamibi
Evaluation of regional myocardial function is a key step in the evaluation of myocardial viability. Indeed, demonstration of persisting function, whether it is normal function or mild hypokinesia, already establishes persistent viability. The issue of residual viability is only pertinent in regions of severe wall motion abnormality such as severe hypokinesia, akinesia or dyskinesia. Analysis of the literature reveals significant confusion in this respect as regions with persistent function have sometimes been classified as 'irreversibly damaged' on the basis of a perfusion defect while persistent viability was clearly evident [34,35]!

Dynamic first pass acquisition is one of the modalities available with Tc-99m Sestamibi to evaluate regional ventricular function [36]. Another approach is to use gated planar or tomographic acquisitions (SPECT) and to analyze these data to extract both global and regional function parameters (global ejection fraction, regional ejection fraction, wall motion, wall thickening) [37]. Such analysis is possible with Tc-99m Sestamibi, while it is not available with thallium-201 due to count rate limitation.

Transient ischemia, occurring during administration at rest or stress but resolved during acquisition, results in a perfusion defect that changes in size between diastole and systole, confirming preserved function. Myocardial infarction or hibernating myocardium results in a persistent perfusion defect that does not change in size during systole. Yet because of the motion of the overall myocardium, persistent perfusion defects may appear to represent a larger percentage of the left ventricle in systole than in diastole.

Several authors have pointed out that evaluation of regional perfusion may be more accurate on the diastolic images than on blurred, ungated images [38]. Patients with stunned myocardium have persisting regional dysfunction despite reperfusion [39]. In these patients, the distribution of perfusion tracers should be normal or near normal, although it remains affected by partial volume effect and resolution recovery factors [40]. Again, evaluation of myocardial perfusion should be more accurate using diastolic images than using ungated images. Demonstration of stunned myocardium in the follow-up of an acute myocardial infarction implies successful reperfusion and potential functional recovery [39].

Clinical experience using Tc-99m Sestamibi as a perfusion tracer

Since its introduction several years ago, Tc-99m Sestamibi has been recognized as a clinically effective perfusion tracer [41–45]. Planar or tomographic techniques can be used but SPECT has been recognized as more sensitive in detecting individual vessel disease while its specificity can be optimized through rigorous quality control.

The diagnostic value of Tc-99m Sestamibi to detect myocardial infarction and myocardial ischemia is at least comparable to thallium-201. Initial experiences by Dilsizian and Rocco have shown a good correlation of qualitative and quantitative uptake of Tc-99m Sestamibi with both the severity of coronary artery stenosis and clinical markers of potential viability [44–45]. Planar scintigraphic uptake in territories supplied by an occluded coronary artery with poor collateral flow was $42 \pm 21\%$, contrasting with $61 \pm 23\%$ (occluded arteries with good collateral flow), $74 \pm 19\%$ (stenosis of 50–99%) and $87 \pm 16\%$ (stenosis < 50%). In patients with previous myocardial infarction, uptake in akinetic regions ($39 \pm 16\%$) was lower than in regions with hypokinetic or normal wall motion ($62 \pm 15\%$). As demonstrated by Gibson *et al.* [46], patency of the infarct-related artery during acute myocardial infarction results in significant defect regression between the acute study and a control 18–48 hours later. Infarct size and severity are larger in the anterior than in the inferior and lateral locations but defect changes are also larger in this location. Defect changes are minimal when the artery remains occluded.

The perfusion defect demonstrated by Tc-99m Sestamibi at discharge is closely related to the level of the left ventricular ejection fraction (LVEF). Significant changes in LVEF values appeared to result from initial stunning or hyperkinesia disappearing at 6 weeks' follow-up [39].

These results contrast with the results of Maublant *et al.* [47], who reported similar perfusion defects in myocardial infarction using thallium-201 or Tc-99m Sestamibi but smaller and fewer defect contrasts using Tc-99m Sestamibi in myocardial ischemia [47]. Similar results have been reported in the experimental animal by Leon *et al.* [48], when studying the effect of short (40 seconds) partial coronary obstructions. Insufficient delay between Tc-99m Sestamibi injection and end of exercise or ischemia may explain these differences. Alternatively, both authors' use of quantification programs optimized for thallium-201 and applied unchanged for Tc-99m Sestamibi might explain these discrepancies.

Clinical experience of the use of Tc-99m Sestamibi to evaluate myocardial Viability

Few reports have analyzed the value of Tc-99m Sestamibi in identifying viable myocardium. As pointed out earlier, experimental studies indicate that viability is required for uptake and retention of Tc-99m Sestamibi while this tracer is released from the infarcted zone, even when it is injected before coronary occlusion [49]. Marzullo *et al.* have published two almost identical papers relating Tc-99m Sestamibi uptake to coronary angiography and wall motion evaluated by echocardiography before and after revascularization [34,35]. Although both studies refer to 14 patients, 9 undergoing coronary artery bypass surgery (CABG) and 5 percutaneous transluminal coronary angioplasty (PTCA), at least some of the patients appear different as the numbers vary slightly between the two studies. In addition, the study published in the *American Journal of Cardiology* (AJC) includes thallium-201 data not presented in the *Journal of Nuclear Medicine* (JNM). The authors have divided their 14 patients into three groups and then analyzed segments rather than patients. In group 2, in segments with normal wall motion but cross-sectional coronary area stenosis of 85 ± 14%, Tc-99m Sestamibi, but not thallium-201, detects a perfusion abnormality at rest with an average uptake of 63 ± 8% of peak activity versus 75 ± 9% and 74 ± 10% for initial and delayed thallium-201. According to the JNM report [35], 28 segments in this group (with normal wall motion) have a peak activity < 55%, a threshold described as below 2.5 SD from the normal mean value and implying 'nonviability', an obvious misclassification (or mislabeling) as these segments had normal wall motion! While this 55% threshold may be adequate to detect a perfusion abnormality, it is obviously inadequate to define nonviable segments. Group 3 patients had thallium-201 (early and late) and Tc-99m Sestamibi peak activity averaging 62 ± 14%, 59 ± 13% and 60 ± 15%, respectively.

The average percent of peak activity of early and delayed thallium-201 and Tc-99m Sestamibi in viable and necrotic segments, defined according to postoperative improvement in wall motion, was 67 ± 12%, 67 ± 9%, and 67 ± 13% versus 53 ± 12%, 46 ± 6% and 48 ± 10%. These data are very similar for thallium-201 and Tc-99m Sestamibi, despite somewhat larger standard deviation values for Tc-99m Sestamibi, likely resulting from the application of background substraction using a program previously developed for thallium-201, even if adjusted for Tc-99m Sestamibi.

The authors claim that Tc-99m Sestamibi is primarily a perfusion agent less reliable than thallium-201 in estimating viability. That conclusion is said to be based on a high rate of false-negative results (false necrotic results!). False-negative results, however, occurred in only 25% of viable segments versus 21% and 14% for thallium-201 (out of 49 segments of group 3, 30 hypokinetic and 19 akinetic). Although the number of false necrotic segments is not given in the AJC paper, they number 7 segments in the JNM paper, selected by the same arbitrary and inadequate 55% uptake threshold for the same average uptake of $46 \pm 5\%$ or $46 \pm 7\%$.

We therefore believe that the conclusions of these articles are unwarranted, based on very few segments and even less patients, using an inadequate arbitrary threshold value ($< 55\%$), applied to many segments in whom the viability was not an issue (normal or hypokinetic wall motion). The authors chose to stress the 'limitations' of Tc-99m Sestamibi rather than to highlight its greater sensitivity to detect the perfusion abnormalities associated with coronary stenosis in patients without wall motion abnormality.

This study also stresses the need for post-revascularization follow-up to define viable segments, keeping in mind that nonviable segments may result from inadequate reperfusion or reperfusion injury. Viability should not be arbitrarily defined or *a priori*. Further quantitative analysis of perfusion imaging should be improved through the use of tomographic imaging, regionally varying thresholds and integral quantification of defect severity.

In another study, Cuocolo *et al.* [50] have compared thallium-201 reinjection and Tc-99m Sestamibi to identify viable myocardium in patients with chronic coronary artery disease. Their group of patients included 20 males with documented coronary artery disease (2 or 3 vessels disease) and left ventricular dysfunction. The ejection fraction ranged from 15–45% (mean $30 \pm 8\%$). However, no functional data nor follow-up information were available in this study. In fact, the presence of increased thallium uptake upon reinjection was arbitrarily considered as the standard for viability. Fifteen segments were analysed per patient for a total of 300 segments. Of these segments, 154 were normal by thallium-201 and Tc-99m Sestamibi; 146 were abnormal. Twenty-four segments had reversible defects by thallium-201 exercise/redistribution and, additionally, after thallium-201 reinjection, partial reversibility was present in 28 segments and complete normalization in 29 segments. In contrast, 43 segments were judged reversible by the Tc-99m Sestamibi exercise/rest protocol.

Several limitations were present in this study. Images were not analyzed quantitatively, although a qualitative uptake score was constructed based on a segmental reading using a 5-point scale. Further, neither functional nor follow-up information was available to independently classify viable and nonviable myocardium and allow retrospective definition of optimal criteria to detect viable myocardium using both tracers. Indeed, these criteria need not be identical for thallium-201 and Tc-99m Sestamibi.

The study of Cuocolo *et al.* [50] suggests different results for both tracers, as thallium-201 reinjection shows more tracer reversibility than Tc-99m Sestamibi. It is, however, impossible to judge from the reported data whether thallium-201 reinjection overestimates viability or whether Tc-99m Sestamibi underestimates it. Experimental data make both alternatives possible and one abstract by Willemart indeed suggests both situations to clinically occur (overestimation of viability by thallium-201 and underestimation of viability by Tc-99m Sestamibi) [51]. Furthermore, the predictive value, especially the positive predictive value, for viability of either FDG or thallium-201 is not better than 75–80% in the literature, making it difficult to use viability prediction as a standard rather than actual follow-up data providing definite proof of viability [52,53].

Bisi *et al.* [54] recently tested the value of Tc-99m Sestamibi imaging during nitrate infusion to predict the outcome of coronary revascularization. In 19 patients with prior myocardial infarction and left ventricular dysfunction, scheduled for PTCA or CABG, rest Tc-99m Sestamibi first pass imaging and perfusion SPECT were performed. A second SPECT study was performed on a separate day, after 15 minutes of nitrate infusion (isosorbide dinitrate 10 mg over 20 minutes). At least 3 months after revascularization, the left ventricular function was assessed with another rest first pass study. In 8 patients, a decrease > 10% in defect size was observed during nitrate infusion and these patients were considered to be responders. In the remaining 11 patients, a > 10% decrease was not observed and they were considered to be non-responders. Baseline left ventricular ejection fraction and defect extent of responders and non-responders were not significantly different. However, after revascularization, the LVEF of responders increased significantly and, also, in this group the defect size decreased significantly. These phenomena were not observed in the non-responders group. The authors therefore concluded that a decrease of the perfusion defect extent in nitrate Tc-99m Sestamibi SPECT versus baseline seems to have a good predictive value for the functional outcome of coronary revascularization. Scoparino *et al.* [55] confirmed the data of Bisi *et al.* [54]. These authors also found Tc-99m Sestamibi imaging after nitrates an accurate test for detection of chronically ischemic dysfunctioning myocardium.

The use of stress/rest protocols to evaluate residual ischemia after myocardial infarction also has the value of predicting functional recovery after revascularization. Benoit *et al.* performed quantitative Tc-99m Sestamibi SPECT studies in 15 patients with recent myocardial infarction before and after revascularization (PTCA or CABG) [56]. Functional recovery was documented by echocardiography. Four of the 15 patients without residual ischemia before revascularization did not improve, while 10 out of 11 patients with residual ischemia after myocardial infarction, demonstrated by Tc-99m Sestamibi, had functional and perfusion improvement during follow-up. Demonstration of residual ischemia after myocardial infarction either by stress testing or by left ventricular unloading therefore provides evidence of jeopardized myocardium capable of benefitting from revascularization, helping to differentiate it from incomplete myocardial infarction without potential improvement.

A number of authors have analyzed the value of Tc-99m Sestamibi for the prediction of viability in conjunction with a metabolic tracer. Altehoefer *et al.* [57] compared the degree of Tc-99m Sestamibi uptake reduction (in percentage of peak activity) to the uptake of FDG normalized to the value in segments of reference normal perfusion. Eighty percent of segments with severe Tc-99m Sestamibi defects (< 30% of peak uptake), 48% of moderate (31–50% of peak uptake) and 31% of mild (> 50% of peak uptake) defects were considered nonviable on the basis of FDG uptake. Normal or near-normal FDG uptake was found in none of the severe defects, in contrast to 29% of moderate and 35% of mild perfusion defects. Although this study lacks follow-up data, it emphasizes the need for quantitative assessment of Tc-99m Sestamibi defect severity rather than a simple descriptive dichotomy (normal/abnormal) to stratify patients and regions according to the probability of viability and recovery.

In a recent report, Soufer *et al.* [58] also compared FDG PET with Tc-99m Sestamibi SPECT imaging. In 36 patients, they analyzed 180 segments and found concordant results in 130 segments. Discordant Tc-99m Sestamibi scar/FDG viable segments were present in 37 patients, 20 of which had segments in the inferior wall. Tc-99m Sestamibi activity in these segments was intermediate between values in viable and nonviable segments (55% of maximum versus 74% and 40%, respectively). The authors concluded that inferior wall viability is understimated by Tc-99m Sestamibi SPECT, probably due to diaphragmatic attenuation artefacts.

Conclusions

It appears from this review that the role of technetium-labeled flow tracers and, in particular, Tc-99m Sestamibi for the evaluation of myocardial viability has not been fully elucidated, as sufficient, properly designed studies are not yet available.

The following points can, however, be stressed from the available data.

1) It is not reasonable to expect that any tracer will accurately separate patients or segments with and without residual viability. Indeed, as jeopardized myocardium is frequently mixed with necrotic areas, it is more likely to expect definition of thresholds indicating probable lack of viability below a threshold and presence of viability above another threshold, while the probability and/or degree of recovery would continuously vary between the two thresholds. This holds true for all tracers and techniques.

2) Using Tc-99m Sestamibi, the primary parameter available for indicating potential viability is its uptake in proportion to blood flow. This is in contrast to thallium-201, where the primary parameter is the extent of redistribution. It would therefore be surprising if similar threshold values could be used with both tracers and, indeed, the experience of those authors attempting to apply similar criteria has not been rewarding.

On the other hand, the biological properties of Tc-99m Sestamibi, lack of uptake and retention in infarcted tissue and depolarized cells, provide optimal ground on which to base diagnosis of lack of viability, when uptake is profoundly depressed and a transient severe reduction in flow can be excluded by a repeated study, preferably with nitrates or using clinical information. Again an adequate threshold needs to be defined. Tc-99m Sestamibi appears superior to thallium in this respect, as evidence from biological and experimental animal studies suggests preserved thallium-201 uptake in severely injured cells and infarcted tissue.

3) Definition of the adequate thresholds requires sophisticated quantitative programs of analysis and preferably the use of SPECT. Indeed, adequate background substraction on planar Tc-99m Sestamibi images remains difficult and the source of data variability.

4) The most difficult differential diagnosis is between reversible chronic dysfunction caused by hibernating myocardium, and non-reversible dysfunction corresponding to incomplete myocardial infarction. The degree of residual stenosis in the artery responsible for the infarct and evidence for residual ischemia in this region should be helpful in that differential diagnosis.

5) Additional parameters of viability available with Tc-labeled flow tracers are to be derived from global and regional ventricular function data through first pass or gated studies.

References

1. Bonow RO, Dilsizian V. Thallium-201 and technetium-99m-sestamibi for assessing viable myocardium. J Nucl Med 1992; 33: 815–8.
2. Willerson JT. Technetium-99m MIBI as a myocardial perfusion agent. Circulation 1990; 82: 1067–9.
3. Machac J. Technetium-99m isonitrile: A perfusion or a viability agent? J Am Coll Cardiol 1989; 14: 1685–8.
4. Beller GA, Ragosta M, Watson DD, Gimple LW. Myocardial thallium-201 scintigraphy for assessment of viability in patients with severe left ventricular dysfunction. Am J Cardiol 1992; 70: 18E–22E.
5. Louie HW, Laks H, Milgalter E, Drinkwater DC Jr, Hamilton MA, Brunken RC et al. Ischemic cardiomyopathy. Criteria for coronary revascularization and cardiac transplantation. Circulation 1991; 84 (5 Suppl): III290–5.
6. Lucas JR, Botvinick EH, Dae MW. Myocardial viability evidence provided by the analysis of left ventricular systolic function. Coronary Artery Dis 1993; 4: 485–94.
7. Grégoire J, Théroux P. Detection and assessment of unstable angina using myocardial perfusion imaging: Comparison between technetium-99m sestamibi SPECT and 12-lead electrocardiogram. Am J Cardiol 1990; 66: 42E–46E.
8. Heyndricks GR, Millard RW, McRitchie RJ, Maroko PR, Vatner SF. Regional myocardial functional and electrophysiological alterations after brief coronary artery occlusion in conscious dogs. J Clin Invest 1975; 56: 978–85.
9. Braunwald E, Kloner RA. The stunned myocardium: Prolonged, post-ischemic ventricular dysfunction. Circulation 1982; 66: 1146–9.
10. Braunwald E, Rutherford JD. Reversible ischemic left ventricular dysfunction: evidence for the 'hibernating myocardium'. J Am Coll Cardiol 1986; 6: 1467–70.
11. Depré CH, Melin JA, Vanoverschelde JL, Borgers M, Wijns W. Assessment of myocardial viability after bypass surgery by pre-operative PET flow-metabolism measurements and ultrastructural analysis of myocardial biopsies [abstract]. Circulation 1993; 88 (4 Suppl I): I199.
12. Rigo P, Murray M, Taylor DR, Weisfeldt ML, Strauss HW, Pitt B. Hemodynamic and prognostic findings in patients with transmural and nontransmural infarction. Circulation 1975; 51: 1064–70.
13. Gropler RJ, Bergmann SR. Flow and metabolic determinants of myocardial viability assessed by positron emission tomography. Coronary Artery Dis 1993; 4: 495–504.

14. Tillisch J, Brunken R, Marshall R, Schwaiger M, Mandelkern M, Phelps M *et al.* Reversibility of cardiac wall-motion abnormalities predicted by positron tomography. N Engl J Med 1986; 314: 884–8.

15. Pierard LA, De Landsheere CM, Berthe C, Rigo P, Kulbertus HE. Identification of viable myocardium by echocardiography during dobutamine infusion in patients with myocardial infarction after thrombolytic therapy: Comparison with positron emission tomography. J Am Coll Cardiol 1990; 15: 1021–31.

16. Baudhuin TH, Melin J, Bol A, Marwick J, Wyns W. Absolute myocardial blood flow and oxygen consumption are maintained in dysfunctional but viable myocardium [abstract]. Circulation 1992; 86 (4 Suppl II): II417.

17. De Silva R, Yamamoto Y, Rhodes CG, Iida H, Nihoyannopoulos P, Davies GJ *et al.* Preoperative prediction of the outcome of coronary revascularization using positron emission tomography. Circulation 1992; 86: 1738–42.

18. Goldstein RA. Rubidium 82 kinetics after coronary occlusion: Temporal relation of net myocardial accumulation and viability in open-chested dogs. J Nucl Med 1986; 27: 1456–61.

19. Wijns W, Baudhuin TH, Bol A, De Pauw M, Cogneau M, Labar D *et al.* Myocardial perfusion and necrosis estimates with potassium-38 in experimental canine myocardial infarction [abstract]. Eur Heart J 1993; 14 (abstract Suppl): 187.

20. Piwnica-Worms D, Kronauge JF, Chiu ML. Uptake and retention of hexakis (2-methoxyisobutyl isonitrile) technetium (I) in cultured chick myocardial cells. Mitochondrial and plasma membrane potential dependence. Circulation 1990; 82: 1826–38.

21. Piwnica-Worms D, Chiu ML, Kronauge JF. Divergent kinetics of 201Tl and 99mTc-SESTAMIBI in cultured chick ventricular myocytes during ATP depletion. Circulation 1992; 85: 1531–41.

22. Sapirstein LA. Regional blood flow by fractional distribution of indicators. Am J Physiol 1958; 193: 161–8.

23. Leppo JA, Meerdink DJ. Comparison of the myocardial uptake of a technetium-labeled isonitrile analogue and thallium. Circ Res 1989; 65: 632–9.

24. Canby RC, Silber S, Pohost GM. Relations of the myocardial imaging agents 99mTc-MIBI and 201TL to myocardial blood flow in a canine model of myocardial ischemic insult. Circulation 1990; 81: 289–96.

25. Meerdink DJ, Leppo JA. Myocardial transport of hexakis (2-methoxy-isobutylisonitrile) and thallium before and after coronary reperfusion. Circ Res 1990; 66: 1738–46.

26. Mousa SA, Cooney JM, Williams SJ. Relationship between regional myocardial blood flow and the distribution of 99mTc-sestamibi in the presence of total coronary artery occlusion. Am Heart J 1990; 119: 842–7.

27. Marshall RC, Leidholdt EM Jr, Zhang DY, Barnett CA. Technetium-99m hexakis 2-methoxy-2-isobutyl isonitrile and thallium-201 extraction, washout, and retention at varying coronary flow rates in rabbit heart. Circulation 1990; 82: 998–1007.

28. Beller GA, Watson DD. Physiological basis of myocardial perfusion imaging with the technetium 99m agents. Semin Nucl Med 1991; 21: 173–81.

29. Melon PG, Beanlands RS, DeGrado TR, Nguyen N, Petry NA, Schwaiger M. Comparison of technetium-99m sestamibi and thallium-201 retention characteristics in canine myocardium. J Am Coll Cardiol 1992; 20: 1277–83.

30. Sinusas AJ, Trautman KA, Bergin JD, Watson DD, Ruiz M, Smith WH *et al.* Quantification of area at risk during coronary occlusion and degree of myocardial salvage after reperfusion with technetium-99m methoxyisobutyl isonitrile. Circulation 1990; 82: 1424–37.

31. Melin JA, Becker LC, Bulkley BH. Differences in Thallium-201 uptake in reperfused and nonreperfused myocardial infarction. Circ Res 1983; 53: 414–9.

32. Sinusas AJ, Watson DD, Cannon JM Jr, Beller GA. Effect of ischemia and postischemic dysfunction on myocardial uptake of technetium-99m-labeled methoxyisobutyl isonitrile and thallium 201. J Am Coll Cardiol 1989; 14: 1785–93.

33. Glover DK, Sansoy V, Ruiz M, Smith WH, Watson DD, Beller GA. Comparison between Tl-

201 and Sestamibi uptake under experimental conditions of sustained low flow and profound systolic dysfunction [abstrat]. Circulation 1993; 88 (4 Suppl I): I198.

34. Marzullo P, Parodi O, Reisenhofer B, Sambuceti G, Picano E, Distante A *et al.* Value of rest thallium-201/technetium-99m sestamibi scans and dobutamine echocardiography for detecting myocardial viability. Am J Cardiol 1993; 71: 166–72.

35. Marzullo P, Sambuceti G, Parodi O. The role of sestamibi scintigraphy in the radioisotopic assessment of myocardial viability. J Nucl Med 1992; 33: 1925–30.

36. Jones RH, Borges-Neto S, Potts JM. Simultaneous measurement of myocardial perfusion and ventricular function during exercise from a single injection of technetium-99m sestamibi in coronary artery disease. Am J Cardiol 1990; 66: 68E–71E.

37. Maisey MN, Mistry R, Sowton E. Planar imaging techniques used with technetium-99m sestamibi to evaluate chronic myocardial ischemia. Am J Cardiol 1990; 66: 47E–54E.

38. Faber TL, Akers MS, Peshock RM, Corbett JR. Three-dimensional motion and perfusion quantification in gated single-photon emission computed tomograms. J Nucl Med 1991; 32: 2311–7.

39. Christian TF, Behrenbeck T, Pellikka PA, Huber KC, Chesebro JH, Gibbons RJ. Mismatch of left ventricular function and infarct size demonstrated by technetium-99m isonitrile imaging after reperfusion therapy for acute myocardial infarction: identification of myocardial stunning and hyperkinesia. J Am Coll Cardiol 1990; 16: 1632–8.

40. Beller GA, Glover DK, Sansoy V, Ruiz M, Smith WH, Watson DD. Effect of resolution of transient ischemic dysfunction on Sestamibi defect severity [abstract]. Circulation 1993; 88 (4 Suppl I): I581.

41. Kiat H, Maddahi J, Roy LT, Van Train K, Friedman J, Resser K *et al.* Comparison of technetium-99m methoxysobutyl isonitrile and thallium-201 for evaluation of coronary artery disease by planar and tomographic methods. Am Heart J 1989; 117: 1–11.

42. Kahn JK, McGhie I, Akers MS, Sils MN, Faber TL, Kulkarni PV *et al.* Quantitative rotational tomography with 201Tl and 99mTC 2-methoxy-isobutyl-isonitrile. A direct comparison in normal individuals and patients with coronary artery disease. Circulation 1989; 79: 1282–93.

43. Maddahi J, Kiat H, Van Train KF, Prigent F, Friedman J, Garcia EV *et al.* Myocardial perfusion imaging with technetium-99m sestamibi SPECT in the evaluation of coronary artery disease. Am J Cardiol 1990; 66: 55E–62E.

44. Dilsizian V, Rocco TP, Strauss HW, Boucher CA. Technetium-99m isonitrile myocardial uptake at rest. I. Relation to severity of coronary artery stenosis. J Am Coll Cardiol 1989; 14: 1673–7.

45. Rocco TP, Dilsizian V, Strauss HW, Boucher CA. Technetium-99m iso-nitrile myocardial uptake at rest. II. Relation to clinical markers of potential viability. J Am Coll Cardiol 1989; 14: 1678–84.

46. Gibson WS, Christian TF, Pellikka PA, Behrenbeck T, Gibbons RJ. Serial tomographic imaging with technetium-99m-sestamibi for the assessment of infarct-related arterial patency following reperfusion therapy. J Nucl Med 1992; 33: 2080–5.

47. Maublant JC, Marcaggi X, Lusson JR, Boire JY, Cauvin JC, Jacob P *et al.* Comparison between thallium-201 and technetium-99m methoxyisobutyl isonitrile defect size in single-photon emission computed tomography at rest, exercise and redistribution in coronary artery disease. Am J Cardiol 1992; 69: 183–7.

48. Leon AR, Eisner RL, Martin SE, Schmarkey LS, Aaron AM, Boyers AS *et al.* Comparison of single-photon emission computed tomographic (SPECT) myocardial perfusion imaging with thallium-201 and technetium-99m sestamibi in dogs. J Am Coll Cardiol 1992; 20: 1612–25.

49. Freeman I, Grunwald AM, Hoory S, Bodenheimer MM. Effect of coronary occlusion and myocardial viability on myocardial activity of technetium-99m-sestamibi. J Nucl Med 1991; 32: 292–8.

50. Cuocolo A, Pace L, Ricciardelli B, Chiariello M, Trimarco B, Salvatore M. Identification of viable myocardium in patients with chronic coronary artery disease: Comparison of thallium-201 scintigraphy with reinjection and technetium-99m-methoxyisobutyl isonitrile. J Nucl Med 1992; 33: 505–11.

51. Willemart B, Melin JA, deKock M, Decoster P, Dereme T, Wijns W. Comparative assessment of myocardial viability with Thallium-201 and Tc 99m-Sestamibi spect imaging [abstract]. J Nucl Med 1992; 33 (5 Suppl): 905–6.
52. Ragosta M, Beller GA, Watson DD, Kaul S, Gimple LW. Quantitative planar rest-redistribution 201Tl imaging in detection of myocardial viability and prediction of improvement in left ventricular function after coronary bypass surgery in patients with severely depressed left ventricular function. Circulation 1993; 87: 1630–41.
53. Schwaiger M, Muzik O. Assessment of myocardial perfusion by positron emission tomography. Am J Cardiol 1991; 67: 35D–43D.
54. Bisi G, Sciagra R, Santoro GM, Briganti V, Pedenovi P, Fazzini PF. Nitrate Sestamibi perfusion imaging: Predictive value for the outcome of coronary revascularization [abstract]. Circulation 1993; 88 (4 Suppl I): I198.
55. Scopinaro F, Banci M, Pagan M. Imaging of viable myocardium with 99mTc Sestamibi injected during nitrate infusion [abstract]. Eur J of Nucl Med 1993; 20 (Suppl): 199.
56. Benoit TH, Pierard L, Foulon J, Berthe C, Pierre-Justin, Rigo P. Quantitative evaluation of tomographic sestamibi scans in the follow-up of patients after myocardial infarction and reperfusion. Eur J Nucl Med 1993; 20 (Suppl): 359.
57. Altehoefer C, Kaiser HJ, Dorr R, Feinendegen C, Beilin I, Uebis R, *et al.* Fluorine-18 deoxyglucose PET for assessment of viable myocardium in perfusion defects in 99mTc-MIBI SPET: A comparative study in patients with coronary artery disease. Eur J Nucl Med 1992; 19: 334–42.
58. Soufer R, Dey HM, Markey J, Ng C, Rich D, Zaret BL. Inferior wall myocardial viability is underestimated on Sestamibi SPECT: Comparison to FDG positron emission tomography [abstract]. Circulation 1993; 88 (4 Suppl I): 199.

5. Delineation of viable myocardium with metabolic imaging

STEVEN R. BERGMANN

Identification of myocardium likely to benefit from pharmacologic, mechanical, or surgical therapies is critical in the care of patients with coronary artery disease. Because more advanced interventional procedures are associated with higher morbidity and mortality, especially in patients with impaired ventricular function, diagnostic approaches that aid in the decision-making process are clearly needed to delineate those patients most likely to derive benefit.

Critical to the discussion that follows are definitions of viable and nonviable myocardium. For the sake of this review, *viable* myocardium refers to areas of dysfunctional that recover functionally after revascularization, whereas *nonviable* myocardium refers to areas that do not recover functionally. Accordingly, definitive delineation of viable from nonviable myocardium can only be made by the sequential evaluation of regional function before and after revascularization [1]. It must be remembered, however, that recanalization can be associated with benefits other than improved contractile function, including relief of angina, improved remodeling, and reduction of arrhythmias [2]. Whether these benefits warrant mechanical or surgical interventions in patients with coronary artery disease in whom nonviable myocardium is identified remains to be determined.

A number of modalities can be used in the diagnostic workup of patients who are being considered for interventional procedures. These include stress testing (either exercise or dobutamine) with electrocardiographic, perfusion, or functional assessments, and are reviewed elsewhere in this monograph. This review will focus on the delineation of viable from nonviable myocardium by the use of metabolic imaging with an emphasis on results achievable with positron emission tomography (PET).

Metabolic basis for assessment of viability

Physiologically, there is a close and intimate relationship between myocardial perfusion, metabolism, and contractile function. The heart is an intrinsically aerobic organ that has a high requirement for adenosine triphosphate (ATP) to fuel contraction. The pattern of substrate use by the heart depends on numerous factors, including arterial substrate and albumin content, neurohumoral

A.S. Iskandrian and E.E. van der Wall (eds): Myocardial viability, 53–70.
© 1994 *Kluwer Academic Publishers.*

conditions, and levels of flow and oxygenation [3–5]. Although the heart can metabolize many different substrates to meet its energy needs, under fasting conditions, 60% to 70% of metabolic needs are met by oxidation of fatty acids and the remainder are met by glycolytic metabolism. After a meal, or with oral or intravenous glucose loading, the increased levels of insulin released result in diminished arterial fatty acid content and increased myocardial glucose use. When flow is limited or when energy demands outstrip substrate supply and/or utilization, oxidation of fatty acid is decreased and utilization of glucose is increased (Figure 5.1). These changes in the pattern of substrate use serve as the basis for delineating myocardium at risk with metabolic imaging.

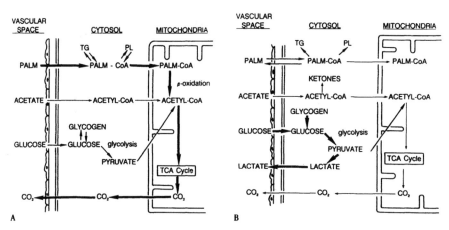

Figure 5.1. Schema of myocardial metabolism under normoxic conditions and during ischemia. A) During normoxia, fatty acids represent the major source for energy production, although the heart can use a variety of other substrates, including glucose, especially after a carbohydrate meal. B) With ischemia, β-oxidation is inhibited and extracted fatty acids are shunted into neutral lipids (triacylglycerides and phospholipids). Backdiffusion is increased as well. Glucose metabolism, both aerobic and anaerobic, is enhanced. Abbreviations: PALM = palmitate; TG = triglyceride; PL = phospholipid; CoA = coenzyme-A; TCA = tricarboxylic acid. (Reproduced with permission, from Bergmannn [8]).

Although the metabolic events that occur with acute coronary occlusion have been extensively studied in experimental preparations, changes that occur with more insidious coronary artery narrowing, as is typically manifest in patients with chronic coronary artery disease, has been more difficult to elucidate precisely. With diminished myocardial perfusion at rest or with stress, myocardial dysfunction can occur. Decreased myocardial function can result in decreased myocardial oxygen use based on diminished demands. It has been hypothesized that such myocardium can remain viable for prolonged periods in a state of 'hibernation'. With more severe levels of ischemia, myocardial viability is compromised and necrosis and infarction can develop. With revascularization, oxidative metabolism recovers in viable myocardium and contractile function is restored, albeit at a slower rate [6,7] dependent on the adequacy of reperfusion and the duration and severity of antecedent ischemia.

Prolonged contractile dysfunction can occur even after full restoration of nutritive perfusion, a phenomenon designated as myocardial stunning. Assessments of myocardial viability have focused on these patterns of flow and substrate utilization.

Positron emission tomography

PET is an advanced imaging approach for delineating regional myocardial perfusion and metabolism [8]. Because of the unique characteristics of positron emission and annihilation to yield two high-energy photons emitted 180° from each other, PET is an intrinsically quantitative approach. In addition, the cyclotron-produced positron-emitting radionuclides (oxygen-15 (^{15}O), nitrogen-13 (^{13}N), carbon-11 (^{11}C), and fluorine-18 (^{18}F)) lend themselves to incorporation into compounds of physiologic interest, including a large number of substrates used normally by the myocardium for energy production. A number of studies have exploited these factors to define the flow and metabolic abnormalities that precede and contribute to functional impairment. While it has not been established definitively that PET is superior to other modalities for clinical decision making, the high specificity and sensitivity of PET and its ability to quantitatively evaluate myocardial perfusion and metabolism in absolute terms (i.e., ml/g/min for flow or μmol/g/min for substrate utilization) using physiologically appropriate mathematical models has provided a template for the evaluation of perfusion and metabolic imaging to define viability.

Assessment of perfusion

Although adequate myocardial perfusion is critical to tissue viability, measurement of myocardial perfusion alone (either by PET or by other approaches) does not permit delineation of viable from nonviable myocardium, in large part because of the complex interrelationship between flow, metabolism, and function. Thus, approaches for delineating myocardial viability solely based on relative or absolute levels of flow per se have not been overly successful [9–11]. Thus, in patients with chronic coronary artery disease, the levels of myocardial perfusion may be decreased in viable myocardium due to 'downregulation', but frequently levels of perfusion at rest are near normal. Moreover, a significant overlap exists. The finding of either normal or reduced perfusion in segments of viable but dysfunctional myocardium suggests that, in some cases, mechanical dysfunction may be a manifestation of myocardial stunning or intermittent demand-induced ischemia rather than hibernation.

More recently, the concept of a perfusable tissue index (PTI) has been introduced to differentiate viable from nonviable myocardium by use of ^{15}O-water [12,13]. Although it has been postulated that the PTI represents the fraction of myocardial tissue that is capable of rapidly exchanging water, recent experimental studies from our laboratory have suggested that it more likely reflects heterogeneity of tissue perfusion [14]. Nonetheless, in a limited number of patients undergoing either angioplasty or coronary artery bypass surgery, PTI has been successful in delineating viable from nonviable myocardium [12,13]. Further studies in a larger number of patients will be necessary to corroborate these findings. However, the use of an index of perfusion for delineation of viability, if proven sensitive and specific, would be rapid and convenient.

Metabolic imaging

Use of 1-^{11}C-palmitate

Because of the central role of fatty acid utilization in myocardial metabolism, initial studies focused on identifying the decreased utilization of fatty acid that occurs early during ischemia. Palmitate, the predominant fatty acid circulating in blood, was labeled in the carbon-1 position with ^{11}C.

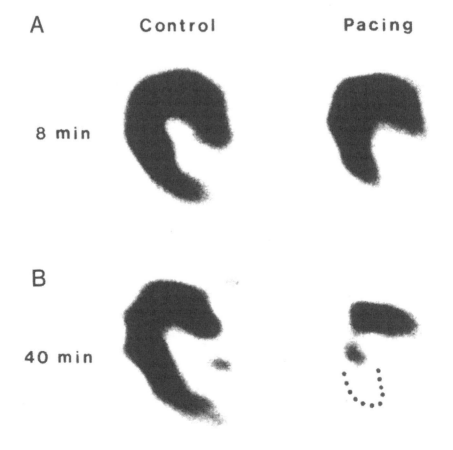

The uptake and release of 1-^{11}C-palmitate have been extensively defined in experimental as well as in clinical studies [15–31]. After initial uptake related to the product of blood flow and extraction, clearance of radioactivity from the heart into blood exhibits two to three components. After initial clearance of tracer not extracted by the myocyte, a rapid component detectable with PET corresponds most directly with rates of mitochondrial beta-oxidation, and a slower component, appearing· later, corresponds with incorporation of fatty acid into neutral lipids (predominantly triglycerides) [17,19,22]. The amount of tracer in each component and the turnover rate can vary based on multiple factors, especially rates of overall oxidative metabolism, blood flow, and oxygenation, and the utilization of fatty acid. With ischemia, the rate of beta-oxidation decreases and is reflected by a decreased clearance of the rapid component of the time-activity curve. This diminished clearance enables

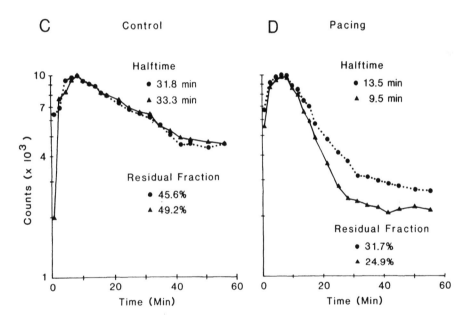

Figure 5.2. Midventricular reconstructions after administration of 1-^{11}C-palmitate under control conditions (left) and during atrial pacing (right) in a patient with 90% stenosis of the left anterior descending coronary artery. Images are oriented with the anterior wall at the upper left, the septum at the upper right, and the lateral wall at the lower left. A) The 8-minute images reflect initial tracer uptake, and B) the 40-minute images reflect clearance of tracer from the myocardium. Uptake is homogenous at rest and during pacing, but clearance becomes heterogeneous with pacing, with greater retention in the anteroseptal myocardium reflective of impaired β-oxidation in myocardium supplied by the stenotic coronary artery.

C) and D) The kinetic curves. Normal myocardium is represented by the triangles and the anteroseptal myocardium (myocardium at risk) by the closed circles. C) Under control circumstances the clearance half-time and residual fractions were similar. D) In contrast, during pacing, the clearance half-time was protracted in the jeopardized region compared with that in normal myocardium. Note, however, that during pacing, overall clearance, thought to be reflective of β-oxidation of fatty acids was increased (i.e., more rapid). This may reflect increased backdiffusion in the poststenotic myocardium. (Reproduced with permission, from Grover-McKay *et al.* [24]).

delineation of viable myocardium in experimental animals with induced coronary artery stenoses studied at rest and again after stress [23]. The changes in clearance rates observed have been shown to be related directly to the decrease in oxidative metabolism and not simply due to the effects of decreased flow [18], confirming the metabolic basis for these findings, which are definable non-invasively with PET. The uptake of palmitate has been useful in defining the salutary effects of reperfusion therapy [27–31].

Grover-McKay *et al.* have demonstrated that kinetics of 1-^{11}C-palmitate uptake and clearance are normal under resting conditions in patients with angiographically documented coronary artery disease and increased (i.e., beta-oxidation of fatty acid was increased) when these patients are subjected to atrial pacing [24]. However, regions supplied by severe stenoses have impaired rates of oxidation, reflected in a flattening of the clearance curve (Figure 5.2) compared with areas supplied by angiographically normal coronary arteries (although it should be noted that the overall rates of clearance are increased compared with those observed under resting conditions).

Despite these encouraging initial observations, a confounding factor in the use of 1-^{11}C-palmitate, which is shared by all long-chain fatty acids used for metabolic imaging is that uptake and utilization by the heart are related to arterial fatty acid concentration; binding of fatty acid to albumin; and levels of perfusion, oxygenation, and the neurohumoral environment, among other factors [19–22]. In human subjects, Schelbert *et al.* demonstrated that changes in arterial fatty acid concentration markedly affected the substrate use of the heart [20,21], and accordingly, the kinetics of myocardial extraction and clearance of 1-^{11}C-palmitate independent of changes in blood flow or oxygenation (Figure 5.3). These findings, coupled with experimental demonstrations [22] that back diffusion of unaltered tracer increases during myocardial ischemia (and would be reflected as enhanced oxidative metabolism), confound the interpretation of myocardial kinetics of 1-^{11}C-palmitate in the setting of ischemia and have resulted in a decline in its use for evaluating myocardial viability.

A number of other fatty acids and fatty acid analogs have been labeled with positron-emitting radionuclides [15]. However, most of the substitutions have been associated with reduced levels of oxidative metabolism and increased retention in triglycerides and other neutral lipids. Thus, these radio-pharmaceuticals predominantly reflect perfusion and uptake of tracer, not oxidative metabolism. This enhances imaging of the heart, but the utility of these tracers for delineating viability is, at present, unclear.

Use of ^{18}F-fluorodeoxyglucose

Increased glucose utilization (both anaerobic and aerobic) relative to flow is one of the metabolic hallmarks of myocardial ischemia [3–5], and imaging with ^{18}F-fluorodeoxyglucose (FDG) was proposed early for use in identification of viable myocardium. This substrate analog traces the initial uptake and phosphor-

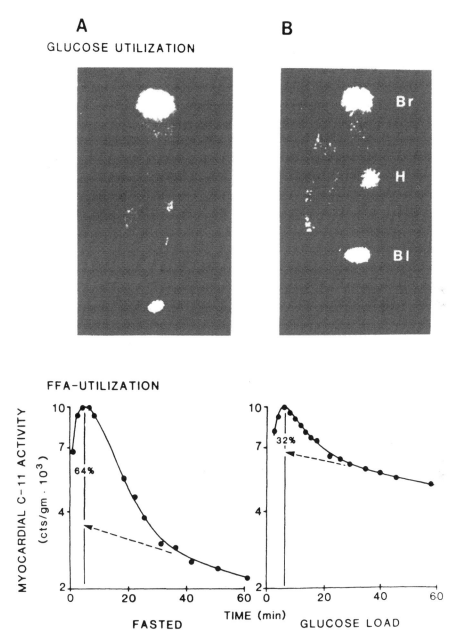

Figure 5.3. Effects of substrate availability on myocardial uptake of ^{18}F-FDG (top) and kinetics of ^{11}C-palmitate (bottom) in the normal human heart. A) Data on the left were obtained after an overnight fast and, B) those on the right, after administration of oral glucose. During fasting conditions, myocardial uptake of ^{18}F-FDG is minimal, but it is enhanced after glucose administration. During fasting, a large proportion of extracted palmitate enters the pool, which turns over rapidly, predominantly representative of β-oxidation. After the glucose load, a smaller proportion enters this pool and the slope of clearance is diminished. This figure illustrates the dependence of the kinetics of these tracers of myocardial metabolism on arterial substrate concentration. Abbreviations: BR = brain; H = heart; BL = bladder. (Reproduced with permission, from Schelbert and Schwaiger [21]).

ylation of glucose. Since the phosphorylated form is not amenable to further metabolism to any extent in the heart, it does not trace further glycolytic metabolism or glycogen synthesis. Most studies in humans are performed after either oral or intravenous glucose loading since the low utilization of glucose under resting circumstances often prevent visualization of the myocardium under fasting conditions because of high blood:tissue ratios [32]. For most imaging procedures, ^{18}F-FDG is administered intravenously, and the myocardium is scanned 45 to 60 minutes after tracer administration – a time sufficient for accumulation of tracer in the heart and clearance of tracer from the blood. Most studies have used qualitative assessments of glucose uptake related to perfusion (assessed with a separate tracer – typically ^{13}N-ammonia, ^{15}O-water, or generator-produced rubidium-82) [33–41]. As discussed below, uptake of glucose by the heart is dependent on multiple factors, including arterial substrate concentration, levels of flow and oxygenation, and neurohumoral environment. In an effort to standardize some of these factors, some investigators have used a euglycemic insulin clamp technique, which although complicated to implement, enhances myocardial glucose utilization [42]. Whether such an approach enhances the detection of viability is unclear. Other investigators advocate performing studies in fasting subjects since this, at times, enhances the identification of ischemic myocardium [43]. Use of ^{18}F-FDG in the diabetic population is problematic. Recent studies have demonstrated good visualization of myocardium in patients with diabetes, although overall utilization of glucose as assessed with ^{18}F-FDG appears to be decreased [44]. It is thus anticipated that future investigations will need to clarify the most appropriate imaging protocol for delineating viability with ^{18}F-FDG.

Marshall et al. [33] first used ^{18}F-FDG to distinguish viable from nonviable myocardium by the demonstration of preserved glycolytic flux in an area of contractile dysfunction. Three general patterns of ^{18}F-FDG uptake related to flow have been described [9–11,33–41] (Figure 5.4) in dysfunctional myocardium: preserved flow and glucose metabolism, reduced flow with preserved glucose metabolism (a flow/metabolism mismatch), and reduced flow and glucose metabolism (a flow/metabolism matched defect). The first two patterns are more typical of regions of myocardial viability, whereas the latter is characteristic of nonviable myocardium. More recently, a pattern of preserved perfusion and reduced glucose metabolism has also been identified that appears to be associated predominantly with viable myocardium when oxidative metabolism is preserved [10,11] (see below). Numerous studies have demonstrated the ability of this approach to define viable from nonviable myocardium [9–11,33–41]. Most have shown that a pattern of enhanced ^{18}F-FDG uptake (with normal or reduced perfusion) is associated with recovery of contractile function after revascularization in 75% to 85% of segments. In regions with concordantly diminished flow and ^{18}F-FDG uptake, 80% to 90% do not improve after revascularization (Table 5.1). Studies from our laboratory have observed lower predictive accuracy [9–11]. Eitzman et al. [45] have demonstrated that patterns of ^{18}F-FDG uptake are strong predictors of future

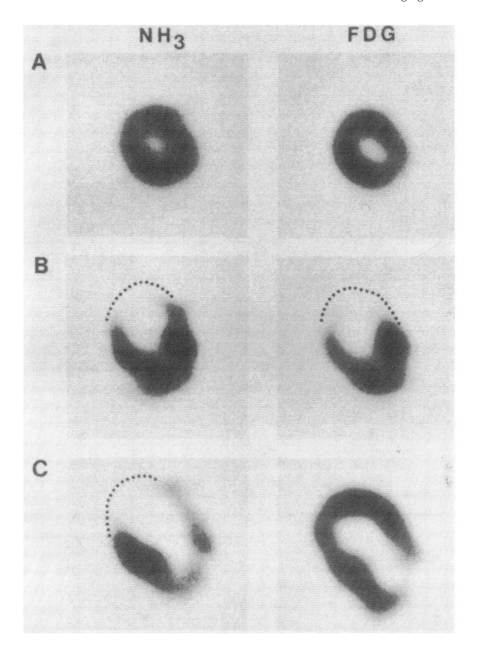

Figure 5.4. A) Distribution of myocardial perfusion evaluated with ^{13}N-ammonia (left) and of glucose metabolism evaluated with ^{18}F-FDG (right) in a normal volunteer showing homogeneous and matching distribution of tracers. B) Tomograms obtained from a patient with myocardial infarction. Blood flow is diminished in the anterior wall (broken lines), associated with a proportional decrease in FDG accumulation and consistent with a pattern of nonviable myocardium. C) Tomograms from a patient in whom myocardial perfusion is diminished in the anterior wall but in whom glucose utilization in the hypoperfused segment is enhanced. This blood flow/metabolism mismatch is reflective of viable myocardium. (Reproduced with permission from Schelbert [34]).

Table 5.1. Accuracy of positron-emission tomography metabolic criteria for detecting viable myocardium

	Subjects, n	Predictive value, %[a] Viable	Predictive value, %[a] Nonviable	Comments
18F-FLUORODEOXYGLUCOSE				
Tillisch et al. [35]	17	85[b]	92[b]	Patients with chronic CAD studied before CABG. Improvement in left ventricular ejection fraction related to number of viable segments present initially.
Tamaki et al. [36]	28	78[b]	80[b]	PET and echocardiographic studies performed before and after CABG. Functional recovery associated with resolution of perfusion and metabolic abnormalities.
Schwaiger et al. [39]	13	50	90	Patients studied 72 h after MI. No thrombolytic agents given or further revascularization procedures implemented.
Piérard et al. [40]	17	55[c]	100[c]	Patients studied 9 days after MI. Functional improvement occurred in 100% of patients with normal flow and metabolism but in only 17% of patients with 'flow-metabolism mismatch'.
Marwick et al. [37]	16	71	76	PET studies performed before and after revascularization. FDG imaging performed after exercise under fasting conditions. Metabolic abnormalities present after revascularization in 29% of viable regions.
Lucignani et al. [38]	14	95	80	Perfusion studies performed with the use of 99mTc-MIBI. FDG studies performed under fasting conditions.
Gropler et al. [11]	34	52[d] 72[e]	81[d] 82[e]	Criteria for viability compared with those with PET and 11C-acetate.
11C-ACETATE				
Gropler et al. [11]	34	67[d] 85[e]	89[d] 87[e]	Criteria for viability compared favorably with those using PET and FDG.
Henes et al. [7]	8	NP	NP	Sequential PET studies performed in patients early after thrombolysis. Functional recovery associated with improvement in oxidative metabolism.
Gropler et al. [9]	11	NP	NP	PET with 11C-acetate and FDG performed before and after CABG or PTCA in patients with recent MI. Maintenance of oxidative metabolism was more reliable than preserved glucose metabolism in determining functional recovery. Metabolic improvement associated with functional recovery.
Gropler et al. [10]	16	NP	NP	PET with 11C-acetate and FDG studies performed in patients with stable CAD before CABG or PTCA. Functional recovery dependent on maintenance of oxidative metabolism and not glucose metabolism.

CABG – coronary artery bypass grafting; CAD – coronary artery disease; FDG – 18F-fluorodeoxyglucose; MI – myocardial infarction; MIBI – sestamibi; NP – not provided; PET – positron-emission tomography; PTCA – percutaneous transluminal coronary angioplasty.

Reproduced with permission, from Gropler and Bergmann [41].

[a] Predictive value = true positives/((true positives + false positives).
[b] Predictive values based on numbers of regions analyzed.
[c] Predictive values based on numbers of patients analyzed.
[d] Predictive values of criteria for mild and moderately dysfunctional segments.
[e] Predictive values of criteria for severely dysfunctional segments.

clinical events. Fifty percent of patients with a pattern indicating viable myocardium, as determined by PET, who did not undergo revascularization suffered myocardial infarction or death within 1 year of the time of the PET scan compared with < 4% of patients with viable myocardium defined metabolically who underwent revascularization. During the same period, death occurred in 5% of patients who did not have viable myocardium as determined by PET (and who did not undergo revascularization).

Although ^{18}F-FDG has been used extensively for identification of viable myocardium with PET, a number of caveats warrant caution. Studies from our laboratory have demonstrated that under fasting conditions, regional disparities in ^{18}F-FDG uptake occur, even in the myocardium of healthy subjects, apparently reflecting regional disparities in the utilization of ^{18}F-FDG by the myocardium [32]. In addition, similar to the case for long-chain fatty acids, accumulation of ^{18}F-FDG is markedly dependent on arterial substrate supply, the pattern of substrate use by the heart, as well as to levels of flow oxygenation (Figures 5.3 and 5.4) [21,32]. Quantitative assessments of glucose utilization by use of ^{18}F-FDG and mathematical modeling to provide an estimate of glucose utilization in μmol/g heart tissue do not appear to improve identification of viable and nonviable myocardium [46]. Some experimental studies have demonstrated that deoxyglucose can accumulate in infarcted tissue [47], and because of the changing patterns of metabolism early after infarction and reperfusion [48], use of ^{18}F-FDG under these circumstances may be more limited than use in evaluating patients with more chronic coronary artery disease. Finally, the use of ^{18}F-FDG by the myocardium does not distinguish between aerobic and anaerobic metabolism [49]. Since it is believed that anaerobic metabolism cannot provide sufficient energy to sustain myocardium for prolonged periods of time, the finding of enhanced ^{18}F-FDG may, under certain circumstances, be ambiguous. Despite these caveats, assessment of viability with ^{18}F-FDG appears promising for delineation of myocardial viability under many circumstances.

Use of ^{11}C-acetate

Because of the problems encountered with the use of labeled long-chain fatty acids and with ^{18}F-FDG, recent efforts have focused on the use of radiopharmaceuticals that quantify levels of overall myocardial oxygen utilization (MVO_2) [50]. There is experimental evidence to suggest that maintenance of oxidative metabolism is a critical factor for viability, and levels of oxygen consumption and recovery of overall oxidative metabolism appear to predict functional recovery after ischemia and reperfusion [6,9–11]. Our group has demonstrated the ability of 1-^{11}C-acetate to delineate overall tricarboxylic acid (TCA) cycle flux and since the TCA cycle is intimately related to oxidative metabolism, the ability of this tracer to delineate overall rates of MVO_2 [50–52]. The use of 1-^{11}C-acetate is predicated on the fact that acetyl-CoA is a central point in the entrance of catabolic metabolism into the mitochondrial

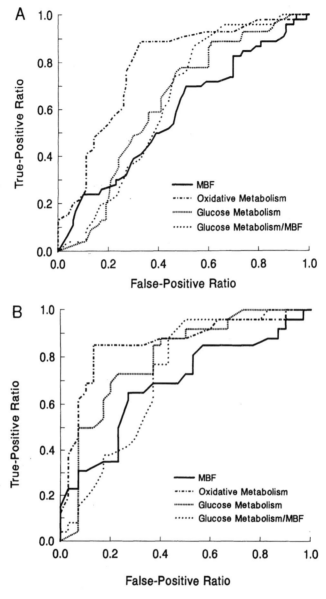

Figure 5.5. Receiver operating characteristic (ROC) curves for the prediction of viable myocardium based on measurements of regional myocardial blood flow (MBF), oxidative metabolism (assessed with 1-^{11}C-acetate), glucose metabolism (assessed with ^{18}F-FDG), and glucose metabolism normalized for MBF in all dysfunctional segments (A) and in severely dysfunctional segments (B) in 34 patients with chronic coronary artery disease. Viability was assessed by sequential functional analysis. Measurements of oxidative metabolism were the most accurate, as reflected by the most left and upward curve. (Reproduced with permission from Gropler et al. [11].)

TCA cycle. Oxidation of acetate to $^{11}CO_2$ (which then effluxes from the myocardium) occurs virtually exclusively in the mitochondria and is directly linked to TCA cycle flux. Monitoring of the rate of efflux of radioactivity from the heart after administration of 1-^{11}C-acetate correlates closely with directly measured MVO_2 over a wide range of physiologic and pathophysiologic conditions. We have further demonstrated that estimates of MVO_2 with 1-^{11}C-acetate are not limited by altered patterns of substrate utilization [53], and we and others have shown that the ability to predict overall regional MVO_2 during ischemia and reperfusion is maintained [51,54].

In clinical studies we demonstrated that levels of oxidative metabolism are low in zones of untreated infarction [55], but recovery of oxidative metabolism to near-normal levels was possible after successful thrombolysis (although the rate of recovery of both oxidative metabolism and of function lagged behind restoration of perfusion) [7]. Recovery of oxidative metabolism was shown to predict the ultimate recovery of function [6,7].

In patients with recent myocardial infarction, as well as in patients with chronic coronary artery disease, levels of oxidative metabolism delineated with 1-^{11}C-acetate predict recovery of function after revascularization [9–11]. The sensitivity and specificity of 1-^{11}C-acetate appear to be superior to those of ^{18}F-FDG (Table 5.1) and superior to those of estimates based on perfusion. In patients with stable coronary artery disease, levels of regional myocardial oxygen consumption delineated with 1-^{11}C-acetate in dysfunctional but viable myocardium are similar to levels observed in normally functioning myocardium and significantly higher than levels observed in nonviable myocardium. In 34 patients with chronic coronary artery disease, near-normal levels of regional MVO_2, as assessed with 1-^{11}C-acetate, were observed in 60 myocardial regions, 40 of which (67%) improved functionally after revascularization procedures. Low levels of regional oxidative capacity were identified in 56 segments, 50 of which did not recover after revascularization, yielding a predictive accuracy of 89%. The rates of positive and negative predictive accuracy were 85% and 87% in regions with severe dysfunction (Figure 5.5).

In our studies, approximately 15% of nonviable segments exhibited increased uptake of ^{18}F-FDG relative to flow that was associated with markedly diminished oxidative metabolism, suggesting that the use of glucose in these regions was primarily anaerobic or due to uptake of ^{18}F-FDG into infarcted or nonmyocardial cells. In contrast, approximately 20% of viable segments exhibited reduced myocardial ^{18}F-FDG uptake, but normal oxidative metabolism, suggesting that nonglycolytic substrate (i.e., fatty acid) was being used for sustained oxidative metabolism [10,11]. It thus appears that maintenance of oxidative metabolism is critical for long-term viability, and predictive of the functional response to revascularization procedures.

Detection of viability with single-photon emitting tracers

A number of investigators have tried to exploit known alterations in myocardial fatty acid metabolism to distinguish viable from nonviable myocardium using single-photon emitting radiotracers (predominantly iodine-123, ^{123}I) and the less expensive and more widely available planar and single-photon emission computed tomographic (SPECT) approaches. Several radiohalogenated radioiodinated fatty acid analogs, including ^{123}I-heptadecanoic acid (IHA), hexadecanoic acid (IHDA), and phenylpentadecanoic acid (IPPA), have been selected for clinical evaluations because their patterns of uptake and clearance are similar to those of 1-^{11}C-palmitate. These patterns do not, however, reflect the same metabolic processes in all circumstances. The myocardial kinetics and clinical use of these compounds have been reviewed recently [56,57].

Zones of myocardial infarction and regions subtended by coronary stenoses are readily detected by patterns of decreased clearance of myocardial radioactivity [56–62]. The use of ^{123}I-HDA has been limited by the appearance of free iodide in the blood, and although correction procedures have been described, they are cumbersome and have not been used extensively. ^{123}I-IPPA shows no release of free radioiodide, but results in the production and release of iodinated benzoic acid by the heart. Although both ^{123}I-HDA and ^{123}I-IPPA have been useful in delineating coronary artery disease and may actually be superior in this respect to thallium-201 (^{201}Tl) [61,62], limited data are available on their utility to define viable from nonviable myocardium. ^{123}I-IPPA has been shown to define regions within zones of persistent defects on ^{201}Tl imaging that have residual ^{18}F-FDG uptake (suggestive of viability although functional outcome was not reported) [61]. Murray *et al.* demonstrated that 73% of dyskinetic segments accumulated ^{123}I-IPPA. Eighty percent of these showed wall motion improvement postoperatively [63]. Nonetheless, it would be anticipated that problems similar to those encountered with 1-^{11}C-palmitate would mitigate the clinical utility of these agents.

Conclusions

PET has provided clinicians with a powerful approach with which to evaluate myocardial perfusion and metabolism. Use of metabolic tracers permits the characterization of the biochemical defects that underlie contractile dysfunction. Nonetheless, data obtained with PET must be interpreted cautiously with a thorough understanding of the metabolic fate of the tracers used and of the multiple factors that can influence tracer kinetics. Recent studies have demonstrated that measures of oxidative metabolism may be the most accurate for defining myocardial viability and thereby identifying those segments likely to benefit from revascularization procedures. Because of the complexity and expense of PET, future studies will need to delineate those circumstances under which PET can and should be used to provide information that cannot be provided by more cost-effective diagnostic approaches. It is likely that PET will continue to provide an enhanced understanding of the pathophysiology of the metabolic patterns that develop during myocardial ischemia and reperfusion and define strategies likely to benefit patients with these disorders. Further correlative studies using single-photon metabolic tracers will be necessary to better define their utility and predictive accuracy.

Acknowledgements

The author thanks Becky Leonard for the preparation of the typescript and Beth Engeszer for the editorial review. Work from the author's lab is funded in part by grants HL-17646 and HL-46895 from National Heart, Lung, and Blood Institute and grant DE-FG02–93ER61659 from the Department of Energy.

References

1. Gropler RJ, Bergmann SR. Myocardial viability – what is the definition? [editorial]. J Nucl Med 1991; 32: 10–2.
2. Becker RC. Late thrombolytic therapy: Mechanism of benefit and potential risk among patients treated beyond 6 hours. Coronary Artery Dis 1993; 4: 293–304.
3. Neely JR, Morgan HE. Relationship between carbohydrate and lipid metabolism and the energy balance of heart muscle. Annu Rev Physiol 1974; 36: 413–59.
4. Liedtke AJ. Alterations of carbohydrate and lipid metabolism in the acutely ischemic heart. Prog Cardiovasc Dis 1981; 23: 321–36.
5. Camici P, Ferrannini E, Opie LH. Myocardial metabolism in ischemic heart disease: Basic principles and application to imaging by positron emission tomography. Prog Cardiovasc Dis 1989; 32: 217–38.
6. Weinheimer CJ, Brown MA, Nohara R, Perez JE, Bergmann SR. Functional recovery after reperfusion is predicated on recovery of myocardial oxidative metabolism. Am Heart J 1993; 125: 939–49.
7. Henes CG, Bergmann SR, Perez JE, Sobel BE, Geltman EM. The time course of restoration of nutritive perfusion, myocardial oxygen consumption, and regional function after coronary thrombolysis. Coronary Artery Dis 1990; 1: 687–96.
8. Bergmann SR. Positron emission tomography of the heart. In Gerson MC (ed): Cardiac Nuclear Medicine. New York: McGraw-Hill 1987; 299–335.
9. Gropler RJ, Siegel BA, Sampathkumaran K, Perez JE, Sobel BE, Bergmann SR *et al.* Dependence of recovery of contractile function on maintenance of oxidative metabolism after myocardial infarction. J Am Coll Cardiol 1992; 19: 989–97.
10. Gropler RJ, Geltman EM, Sampathkumaran K, Perez JE, Moerlein SM, Sobel BE *et al.* Functional recovery after coronary revascularization for chronic coronary artery disease is dependent on maintenance of oxidative metabolism. J Am Coll Cardiol 1992; 20: 569–77.
11. Gropler RJ, Geltman EM, Sampathkumaran K, Perez JE, Schechtman KB, Conversano A *et al.* Comparison of carbon-11-acetate with fluorine-18-fluorodeoxyglucose for delineating viable myocardium by positron emission tomography. J Am Coll Cardiol 1993; 22: 1587–97.
12. Yamamoto Y, de Silva R, Rhodes CG, Araujo LI, Iida H, Recharia E *et al.* A new strategy for the assessment of viable myocardium and regional myocardial blood flow using ^{15}O-water and dynamic positron emission tomography. Circulation 1992; 86: 167–78.
13. de Silva R, Yamamoto Y, Rhodes CG, Iida H, Nihoyannopoulos P, Davies GJ *et al.* Preoperative prediction of the outcome of coronary revascularization using positron emission tomography. Circulation 1992; 86: 1738–42.
14. Herrero P, Staudenerz A, Walsh JF, Gropler RJ, Bergmann SR. Heterogeneity of myocardial perfusion provides the physiological basis of 'perfusable tissue index'. J Nucl Med. In press.

68 *S.R. Bergmann*

15. Lerch RA, Bergmann SR, Sobel BE. Delineation of myocardial fatty acid metabolism with positron emission tomography. In Bergmann SR, Sobel BE (eds): Positron Emission Tomography of the Heart. Mount Kisco: Futura 1992; 129–52.
16. Weiss ES, Hoffman EJ, Phelps ME, Welch MJ, Henry PD, Ter-Pogossian MM *et al.* External detection and visualization of myocardial ischemia with ^{11}C-substrates *in vivo* and *in vitro.* Circ Res 1976; 39: 24–32.
17. Schön HR, Schelbert HR, Robinson G, Najafi A, Huang SC, Hansen H *et al.* C-11 labeled palmitic acid for the noninvasive evaluation of regional myocardial fatty acid metabolism with positron-computed tomography. I. Kinetics of C-11 palmitic acid in normal myocardium. Am Heart J 1981; 103: 532–47.
18. Lerch RA, Bergmann SR, Ambos HD, Welch MJ, Ter-Pogossian MM, Sobel BE. Effect of flow-independent reduction of metabolism on regional myocardial clearance of ^{11}C-palmitate. Circulation 1982; 65: 731–8.
19. Schelbert HR, Henze E, Schon HR, Keen R, Hansen H, Selin C *et al.* C-11 palmitate for the noninvasive evaluation of regional myocardial fatty acid metabolism with positron computed tomography. III. *In vivo* demonstration of the effects of substrate availability on myocardial metabolism. Am Heart J 1983; 105: 492–504.
20. Schelbert HR, Henze E, Sochor H, Grossman RG, Huang SC, Bario JR *et al.* Effects of substrate availability on myocardial C-11 palmitate kinetics by positron emission tomography in normal subjects and patients with ventricular dysfunction. Am Heart J 1986; 111: 1055–64.
21. Schelbert HR, Schwaiger M. PET studies of the heart. In Phelps ME, Mazziotta JC, Schelbert HR (eds): Positron Emission Tomography and Autoradiography: Principles and Applications for the Brain and Heart. New York: Raven Press 1986; 581–661.
22. Fox KA, Abendschein DB, Ambos HD, Sobel BE, Bergmann SR. Efflux of metabolized and nonmetabolized fatty acid from canine myocardium. Implications for quantifying myocardial metabolism tomographically. Circ Res 1985; 57: 232–43.
23. Lerch RA, Ambos HD, Bergmann SR, Welch MJ, Ter-Pogossian MM, Sobel BE. Localization of viable, ischemic myocardium by positron-emission tomography with ^{11}C-palmitate. Circulation 1981; 64: 689–99.
24. Grover-McKay M, Schelbert HR, Schwaiger M, Sochor H, Guzy PM, Krirokapich J *et al.* Identification of impaired metabolic reserve by atrial pacing in patients with significant coronary artery stenosis. Circulation 1986; 74: 281–92.
25. Weiss ES, Ahmed SA, Welch MJ, Williamson JR, Ter-Pogossian MM, Sobel BE. Quantification of infarction in cross sections of canine myocardium *in vivo* with positron emission transaxial tomography and ^{11}C-palmitate. Circulation 1977; 55: 66–73.
26. Ter-Pogossian MM, Klein MS, Markham J, Roberts R, Sobel BE. Regional assessment of myocardial metabolic integrity *in vivo* by positron-emission tomography with ^{11}C-labeled palmitate. Circulation 1980; 61: 242–55.
27. Bergmann SR, Lerch RA, Fox KA, Ludbrook PA, Welch MJ, Ter-Pogossian MM *et al.* Temporal dependence of beneficial effects of coronary thrombolysis characterized by positron tomography. Am J Med 1982; 73: 573–81.
28. Bergmann SR, Fox KA, Ter-Pogossian MM, Sobel BE, Collen D. Clot-selective coronary thrombolysis with tissue-type plasminogen activator. Science 1983; 220: 1181–3.
29. Knabb RM, Rosamond TL, Fox KA, Sobel BE, Bergmann SR. Enhancement of salvage of reperfused ischemic myocardium by diltiazem. J Am Coll Cardiol 1986; 8: 861–71.
30. Knabb RM, Bergmann SR, Fox KA, Sobel BE. The temporal pattern of recovery of myocardial perfusion and metabolism delineated by positron emission tomography after coronary thrombolysis. J Nucl Med 1987; 28: 1563–70.
31. Sobel BE, Geltman EM, Tiefenbrunn AJ, Jaffe AS, Spadaro JJ Jr, Ter-Pogossian MM *et al.* Improvement of regional myocardial metabolism after coronary thrombolysis induced with tissue-type plasminogen activator or streptokinase. Circulation 1984; 69: 983–90.
32. Gropler RJ, Siegel BA, Lee KJ, Moerlein SM, Perry DJ, Bergmann SR *et al.* Nonuniformity in myocardial accumulation of fluorine-18-fluorodeoxyglucose in normal fasted humans. J Nucl Med 1990; 31: 1749–56.

33. Marshall RC, Tilisch JH, Phelps ME, Huang SC, Carson R, Henze E *et al.* Identification and differentiation of resting myocardial ischemia and infarction in man with positron computed tomography, ^{18}F-labeled fluorodeoxyglucose, and N-13-ammonia. Circulation 1983; 67: 766–78.

34. Schelbert HR. Current status and prospects of new radionuclides and radiopharmaceuticals for cardiovascular nuclear medicine. Semin Nucl Med 1987; 17: 145–81.

35. Tillisch J, Brunken R, Marshall R, Schwaiger M, Mandelkern M, Phelps M *et al.* Reversibility of cardiac wall-motion abnormalities predicted by positron tomography. N Engl J Med 1986; 314: 884–8.

36. Tamaki N, Yonekura Y, Yamashita K, Saji H, Magata Y, Senda M *et al.* Positron emission tomography using fluorine-18-deoxyglucose in evaluation of coronary artery bypass grafting. Am J Cardiol 1989; 64: 860–5.

37. Marwick TH, MacIntyre WJ, Lafont A, Nemec JJ, Salcedo EE. Metabolic responses of hibernating and infarcted myocardium to revascularization. A follow-up study of regional perfusion, function, and metabolism. Circulation 1992; 85: 1347–53.

38. Lucignani G, Paolini G, Landoni C, Zuccari M, Paganelli G, Galli L *et al.* Presurgical identification of hibernating myocardium by combined use of technetium-99m hexakis 2-methoxyisobutylisonitrile single photon emission tomography and fluorine-18 fluoro-2-deoxy-D-glucose positron emission tomography in patients with coronary artery disease. Eur J Nucl Med 1992; 19: 874–81.

39. Schwaiger M, Brunken R, Grover-McKay M, Krivokapich J, Child J, Tillisch JH *et al.* Regional myocardial metabolism in patients with acute myocardial infarction assessed by positron emission tomography. J Am Coll Cardiol 1986; 8: 800–8.

40. Píerard LA, De Landsheere CM, Berthe C, Rigo P, Kulbertus HE. Identification of viable myocardium by echocardiography during dobutamine infusion in patients with myocardial infarction after thrombolytic therapy: Comparison with positron emission tomography. J Am Coll Cardiol 1990; 15: 1021–31.

41. Gropler RJ, Bergmann SR. Flow and metabolic determinants of myocardial viability assessed by positron-emission tomography. Coronary Artery Dis 1993; 4: 495–504.

42. Knuuti MJ, Nuutila P, Ruotsalainen U, Saraste M, Harkonen R, Akonen A *et al.* Euglycemic hyperinsulinemic clamp and oral glucose load in stimulating myocardial glucose utilization during positron emission tomography. J Nucl Med 1992; 33: 1255–62.

43. Tamaki N, Yonekura Y, Kawamoto M, Magata Y, Sasayama S, Takahashi N *et al.* Simple quantification of regional myocardial uptake of fluorine-18-deoxyglucose in the fasting condition. J Nucl Med 1991; 32: 2152–7.

44. Voipio-Pulkki LM, Nuutila P, Knuuti MJ, Ruotsalainen U, Haaparanta M, Teras M *et al.* Heart and skeletal muscle glucose disposal in type 2 diabetic patients as determined by positron emission tomography. J Nucl Med 1993; 34: 2064–7.

45. Eitzman D, Al-Aouar Z, Kanter HL, vom Dahl J, Kirsh M, Deet GM *et al.* Clinical outcome of patients with advanced coronary artery disease after viability studies with positron emission tomography. J Am Coll Cardiol 1992; 20: 559–65.

46. Knuuti MJ, Nuutila P, Ruotsalainen U, Teras M, Saraste M, Harkonen R *et al.* The value of quantitative analysis of glucose utilization in detection of myocardial viability by PET. J Nucl Med 1993; 34: 2068–75.

47. Sebree L, Bianco JA, Subramanian R, Wilson MA, Swanson D, Hegge I *et al.* Discordance between accumulation of C-14 deoxyglucose and Tl-201 in reperfused myocardium. J Mol Cell Cardiol 1991; 23: 603–16.

48. Buxton DB, Schelbert HR. Measurement of regional glucose metabolic rates in reperfused myocardium. Am J Physiol 1991; 261: H2058–68.

49. Schwaiger M, Neese RA, Araujo L, Wijns W, Wisneski JA, Sochor H *et al.* Sustained nonoxidative glucose utilization and depletion of glycogen in reperfused canine myocardium. J Am Coll Cardiol 1989; 13: 745–54.

50. Bergmann SR, Sobel BE. Quantification of regional myocardial oxidative utilization by positron emission tomography. In Bergmann SR, Sobel BE (eds): Positron Emission Tomography of the Heart. Mount Kisco: Futura 1992; 209–29.

51. Brown M, Marshall DR, Sobel BE, Bergmann SR. Delineation of myocardial oxygen utilization with carbon-11 labeled acetate. Circulation 1987; 76: 687–96.
52. Brown MA, Myears DW, Bergmann SR. Noninvasive assessment of canine myocardial oxidative metabolism with carbon-11 acetate and positron emission tomography. J Am Coll Cardiol 1988; 12: 1054–63.
53. Brown MA, Myears DW, Bergmann SR. Validity of estimates of myocardial oxidative metabolism with carbon-11 acetate and positron emission tomography despite altered patterns of substrate utilization. J Nucl Med 1989; 30: 187–93.
54. Armbrecht JJ, Buxton DB, Schelbert HR. Validation of [1-^{11}C]acetate as a tracer for noninvasive assessment of oxidative metabolism with positron emission tomography in normal, ischemic, postischemic, and hyperemic canine myocardium. Circulation 1990; 81: 1594–605.
55. Walsh MN, Geltman EM, Brown MA, Henes CG, Weinheimer CJ, Sobel BE et al. Noninvasive estimation of regional myocardial oxygen consumption by positron emission tomography with carbon-11 acetate in patients with myocardial infarction. J Nucl Med 1989; 30: 1798–808.
56. Antar MA. Radiopharmaceuticals for studying cardiac metabolism. Int J Rad Appl Instrum [B] 1990; 17: 103–28.
57. Sochor H, Czernin J, Schelbert HR. Metabolic imaging with single-photon emitting tracers. In Marcus ML, Schelbert HR, Skorton DJ, Wolf GL (eds): Cardiac Imaging: A Companion to Braunwald's-Heart Disease. Philadelphia: Saunders 1991; 1085–96.
58. van der Wall EE, Den Hollander W, Heidendal GAK, Westera G, Majid PA, Roos JP. Dynamic myocardial scintigraphy with ^{123}I-labeled free fatty acids in patients with myocardial infarction. Eur J Nucl Med 1981; 6: 383–9.
59. van der Wall EE, Heidendal GAK, den Hollander W, Westera G, Roos JP. Metabolic myocardial imaging with ^{123}I-labeled heptadecanoic acid in patients with angina pectoris. Eur J Nucl Med 1981; 6: 391–6.
60. Roesler H, Hess T, Weiss M, Noelpp U, Mueller G, Hoeflin F et al. Tomoscintigraphic assessment of myocardial metabolic heterogeneity. J Nucl Med 1983; 24: 285–96.
61. Henrich MM, Vester E, von der Lohe E, Herzog H, Simon H, Kuikka JT et al. The comparison of 2-^{18}F-2-deoxyglucose and 15-(ortho-^{123}I-phenyl)-pentadecanoic acid uptake in persisting defects on thallium-201 tomography in myocardial infarction. J Nucl Med 1991; 32: 1353–7.
62. Hansen CL, Corbett JR, Pippin JJ, Jansen DE, Kulkarni PV, Ugolini V et al. Iodine-123 phenylpentadecanoic acid and single photon emission computed tomography in identifying left ventricular regional metabolic abnormalities in patients with coronary heart disease: Comparison with thallium-201 myocardial tomography. J Am Coll Cardiol 1988; 12: 78–87.
63. Murray G, Schad N, Ladd W, Allie D, van der Zwaag R, Avet P et al. Metabolic cardiac imaging in severe coronary disease: Assessment of viability with iodine-123-iodophenylpentadecanoic acid and multicrystal gamma camera, and correlation with biopsy. J Nucl Med 1992; 33: 1269–77.

6. Echocardiographic assessment of myocardial viability

SANJIV KAUL

Introduction

Before we discuss the echocardiographic methods for assessing myocardial viability, it is important to define the clinical settings where the assessment of myocardial viability is an issue: *regional or global left ventricular dysfunction in the context of coronary artery disease.* One such clinical situation is where myocardial blood flow is reduced on a chronic basis without necessarily having any previous infarction (Figure 6.1A), while another is acute myocardial infarction or ischemia where regional myocardial blood flow has either been fully restored or is still significantly diminished (Figure 6.1B and C). The terms 'hibernating' [1] and 'stunned' [2] myocardium have been used to describe some of these conditions, but since they often coexist (such as an acute infarction in the setting of chronically reduced myocardial blood flow), such terminology should be used with considerable caution. It is clinically more relevant to understand flow-function relations in individual myocardial segments in individual patients rather than characterize patients using terminologies which may or may not accurately define their particular condition.

As indicated above, the assessment of myocardial viability has meaning only in the context of significant coronary artery disease where a revascularization procedure, if indicated, is likely to improve regional and hence global function. If left ventricular function is reduced consequent to other conditions, such as nonischemic cardiomyopathy, determination of myocardial viability is a moot point since in such situations myocardial blood flow and function cannot be improved by revascularization.

Techniques such as positron emission tomography and single-photon imaging have been used to assess myocardial viability because of their ability to either demonstrate ongoing metabolic activity in dysfunctional myocardial cells (positron emission tomography) [3] or indicate intact cell membrane (thallium-201) [4, 5] or mitochondrial (sestamibi) [6] function in such cells. Two-dimensional echocardiography, on the other hand, can be used to assess myocardial viability either by determining regional myocardial function (wall thickening and motion) at rest or during pharmacologic intervention or by assessing microvascular blood flow (contrast echocardiography), or by assessing both. This review will discuss the role of these approaches for the assessment of myocardial viability. Emphasis will be placed on experimental

A.S. Iskandrian and E.E. van der Wall (eds): Myocardial viability, 71–102.
© 1994 *Kluwer Academic Publishers.*

COMMON CLINICAL SCENARIOS WHERE REGIONAL
FUNCTION IS REDUCED BUT THE MYOCARDIUM MAY BE VIABLE

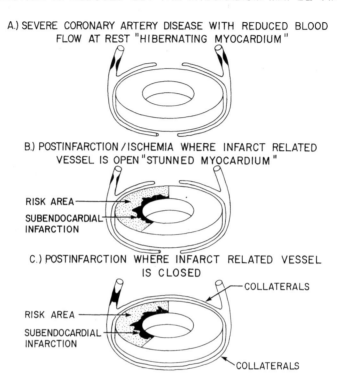

Figure 6.1. Some models of coronary artery disease where myocardial viability is an important clinical issue: A) Persistent chronic reduction in anterograde flow with persistent reduction in regional function. B) Infarction where resting anterograde blood flow has been restored but function is still reduced. C) Occlusion of the infarct-related artery where perfusion is still present via collaterals. Combination of these models can also co-exist within individual patients and individual segments in the same patient. See text for details.

data to explain the basis of the use of echocardiography for this purpose and relevant clinical studies will be discussed.

Assessment of regional function

Flow-function relations in the normal myocardium

The relation between regional wall thickening and anterograde myocardial blood flow in the non-infarcted, non-postischemic, canine myocardium characterized with the use of quantitative two-dimensional echocardiography is depicted in Figure 6.2 [7]. In the range of normal to acutely reduced blood flow (≤ 1 ml/min/g), the relation is almost linear; that is, wall thickening diminishes

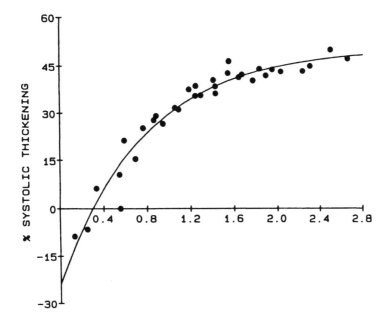

Figure 6.2. The flow-function relation in anesthetized open-chest dogs whose left anterior descending coronary artery was selectively cannulated. The anterograde transmural blood flow (ml/min/g) is measured using radiolabeled microspheres (*x*-axis) and systolic wall thickening (%) is measured using quantitative two-dimensional echocardiography (*y*-axis). The relationship is exponential via a wide range of flows. See text for details. From Kaul *et al.* [17].

linearly with reduction in flow; the lower the flow, the less the wall thickening. Thickening is abolished when transmural blood flow declines to approximately 30% of normal (0.3 ml/min/g) and wall thinning occurs at blood flows below this level. As can be noted from Figure 6.2, when regional blood flow is selectively increased to levels above normal, wall thickening increases in an exponential manner (50% increase at 2.5-fold increase in flow) with no further increase in thickening occurring above flows of 2.5 ml/min/g.

Most of the thickening noted in the myocardium occurs as a consequence of thickening of the endocardium [8–11]. Under normal conditions, the mid-myocardium contributes only a modest amount to overall wall thickening, while the epicardial one-third contributes only minimally to wall thickening. This phenomenon is depicted graphically in Figure 6.3 where sutures were placed to demarcate different layers within the myocardial wall of a beating canine heart. On M-mode echocardiography, it is clear that during systole the myocardial layers on the inner aspect of the wall thicken significantly more than those on the outer aspect [8]. Thus, ischemia or infarction of just the endocardium can lead to a significant diminution of wall thickening at rest.

Thickening of the normal myocardium can be augmented in the presence of catecholamines (such as during exercise or dobutamine infusion) [12]. Although

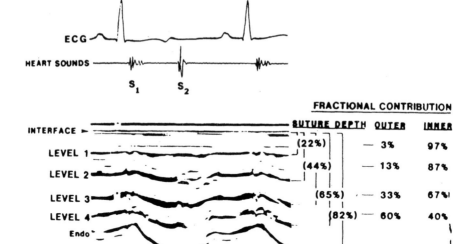

Figure 6.3. Example of M-mode echocardiographic tracing where sutures have been placed within the myocardium at various depths. The excursion of each suture during systole indicates the amount of thickening between that suture and the endocardium (Level 4) or between that suture and the next (Levels 1 to 4). Contribution of the different myocardial layers to total wall thickening decreases as one moves from the endocardium to the epicardium. See text for details. From Myers *et al.* [8], with permission of the American Heart Association.

this increased thickening of the normal myocardium is primarily due to the inotropic effect of the catecholamines, it is also associated with a concomitant increase in myocardial blood flow which reflects increased myocardial oxygen consumption during increased thickening [12]. At high heart rates (above 150 beats/min), the chronotropic effects of catecholamines (Bowditch effect) also contributes some to the increased wall thickening [13]. The effect of upright exercise on the loading conditions of the heart also results in changes in left ventricular cavity size and apparent wall excursion. The vasodilatory effects of dobutamine [14] also causes a reduction in left ventricular chamber size. These phenomena should be kept in mind while performing regional function analysis during exercise or dobutamine echocardiography.

As shown in Figure 6.2, selective increase in myocardial blood flow above normal (> 1 ml/min/g), without altering the inotropic and chronotropic state of the heart and, also, without changing systemic hemodynamics, results in a modest increment in regional wall thickening and can be explained by the erectile nature of the myocardium (Gregg phenomenon) [15]. This phenomenon, however, tapers off at flows greater than 2.5-fold of normal. Some of the increased wall thickening noted during exercise or dobutamine can also be attributed to this effect, which may also explain the increased myocardial thickening noted during adenosine or dipyridamole infusion. Changes in the loading conditions of the heart, such as decreased afterload may also contribute to changes in wall motion and left ventricular size seen during the intravenous infusion of these smooth muscle vasodilators. Lack of increase in wall thickening in myocardial beds subserved by flow-limiting lesions may explain the basis of using these drugs for the detection of coronary artery disease. Frank ischemia (reduction in flow during infusion of the drug when baseline flow is normal) is more likely to occur due to 'coronary steal' seen in the setting of multivessel disease and abundant collateral vessels.

Regional function in the presence of myocardial infarction where the infarct-related artery is occluded

In a set of experiments performed in dogs where the coronary artery was occluded and regional function was assessed with two-dimensional echocardiography 2 days later, complete loss of wall thickening was noted in dogs with infarctions involving 20% or greater of the wall thickness [16]. Function was retained when infarction involved less than 20% of the wall thickness, with better function associated with infarctions involving smaller portions of the wall (Figure 6.4). *Any retained wall thickening at rest during an infarction, therefore, signifies the presence of viable myocardium.* In contrast, however, no consistent relation was found between wall thinning and the transmural extent of infarction. That is, beyond the 20% threshold, larger transmural infarcts did not

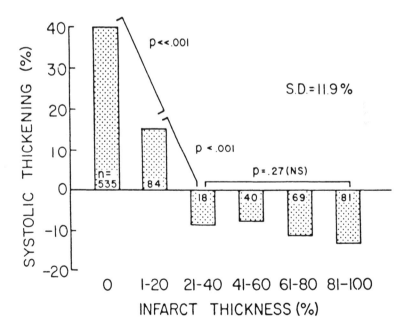

Figure 6.4. Relation between the transmural extent of infarction (*x*-axis) and regional wall thickening (*y*-axis) in dogs with 48 hours of coronary occlusion with no reflow. Some thickening is maintained as long as ≤ 20% of the transmural thickness is infarcted. Infarctions involving > 20% thickness of the myocardium results in wall thinning. There is no relation between percent wall thinning and the transmural extent of infarction. See text for details. From Liberman *et al.* [16], with permission of the American Heart Association.

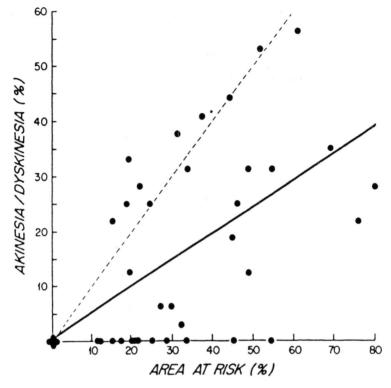

Figure 6.5. Relation between risk area (*x*-axis) and circumferential extent of akinesia (*y*-axis) in dogs with coronary occlusion. It is evident that akinesia is not noted until the risk area is ≥ 12% of the myocardial short axis slice. See text for details. From Kaul *et al.* [17], with permission of the American College of Cardiology.

necessarily result in greater wall thinning. *Loss of resting wall thickening in the context of infarction, therefore, does not preclude the presence of viable myocardium within the infarct bed.*

In the clinical situation, since at times it is easier to assess regional wall motion than wall thickening, it is also important to consider the relation between wall motion and infarct size. One of the factors that determines whether wall motion is abnormal in infarction (or ischemia) is the circumferential extent of infarction (or ischemia). An infarction (or ischemia) involving only a small portion of the left ventricular circumference (< 12%) may not result in loss of regional function due to the tethering effect of adjacent normal myocardium (Figure 6.5) [17] which will 'pull-in' the infarcted or ischemic tissue. Another factor is the loading condition of the left ventricle. Changes in load (such as acute mitral regurgitation) may cause motion of infarcted (or ischemic) myocardium [18] and may result in misinterpretation of the viability status of the myocardium. Also, cardiac translation that occurs with respiration and the change in left ventricular geometry that can occur with infarction or ischemia are far less likely to affect the quantification of regional

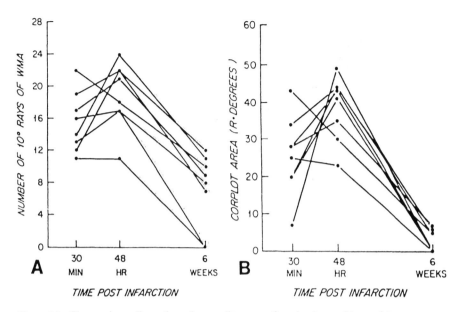

Figure 6.6. Change in wall motion abnormality over time in dogs with persistent coronary occlusion. A) Change in the circumferential extent of any abnormal wall motion. B) Change in the circumferential extent of only dyskinesia. From Gibbons *et al.* [20], with permission of the American Heart Association.

wall thickening than wall motion [19]. It is for these reasons that, whenever possible, it is better to assess regional thickening rather than regional motion.

In dogs with infarction who have been followed for 6 weeks, it has been shown that both the degree and circumferential extent of regional left ventricular dysfunction decrease over time despite a persistently occluded infarct-related artery (Figure 6.6) [20]. These findings are also frequently seen in patients with acute myocardial infarction, especially those with inferior infarction, and implies the occurrence of two phenomena. First, despite significant transmural ischemia, portions of the myocardium do not undergo necrosis during acute coronary occlusion. It is well known, for instance, that necrosis occurs only within regions receiving < 20–30% of baseline flow. If there is abundant residual collateral-derived blood flow within the infarct bed, islands of myocardial tissue will escape necrosis [21]. Second, due to metabolic needs of these viable cells, especially during exercise, further maturation of collateral vessels occurs over time resulting in an increase in resting blood flow and improved regional function.

Regional function in the presence of myocardial infarction where the infarct-related artery is patent

When myocardium is rendered ischemic and then adequate resting flow is reestablished, regional function does not return immediately to normal [1, 22].

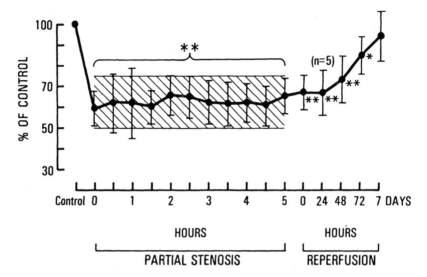

Figure 6.7. Time-course of improvement in regional function after 1 hour of ischemia in a dog. There was no necrosis and full recovery in function occurred in 7 days. This is an example of the pure 'stunned myocardium'. From Matsuzaki *et al.* [23], with permission from the American Heart Association.

In the absence of infarction, the time taken for regional function to recover is influenced by the duration of coronary occlusion; longer occlusions result in more prolonged periods of dysfunction. This phenomenon of post-ischemic myocardial dysfunction has been termed the 'stunned myocardium' [1] and is graphically depicted in Figure 6.7 where it took 7 days for regional function to fully recover after 5 hours of ischemia in the dog [23]. 'Stunned myocardium', however, implies lack of necrosis within the ischemic bed which is uncommon in the clinical setting. Clinical examples of the pure 'stunned myocardium' are post-exercise myocardial dysfunction occasionally noted in patients undergoing stress testing [24–26], in those with unstable angina [27, 28], and after coronary angioplasty [28].

The most common scenario for postischemic dysfunction, however, is in acute myocardial infarction where reperfusion has been established either pharmacologically or mechanically (Figure 6.1, panel A) [29–34]. Despite significant residual coronary stenosis, resting regional myocardial blood flow is normal or near normal in most of these patients. Unlike the canine model of 'stunned myocardium', however, where there is no myocardial necrosis, in patients, variable amounts of necrosis coexist with post-ischemic dysfunction. In these patients, like the canine model, *the duration of myocardial dysfunction is related to the duration of ischemia* (coronary occlusion in this case), but *the degree of ultimate functional recovery is related to the amount and location of myocardial necrosis.* In patients with negligible necrosis as a result of very early (within one hour of onset of coronary occlusion) restoration of flow, complete recovery in function may occur [29]; in most patients, however, the recovery in function is incomplete [30–33].

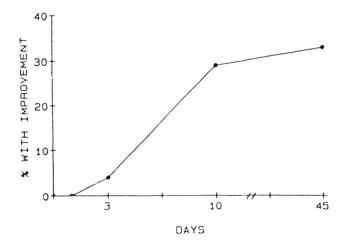

Figure 6.8. Percent of patients (*y*-axis) demonstrating improvement in regional function over time (*x*-axis) after receiving intravenous streptokinase within 4 hr of chest pain. Most patients showed recovery in function between 3 and 10 days. See text for details. From Touchstone *et al.* [31], with permission of the American College of Cardiology.

Figure 6.8 depicts the percent of patients with acute myocardial infarction demonstrating recovery in regional function after reperfusion therapy [31]. All patients received 1.5 million IU of intravenous streptokinase within 4 hours after onset of chest pain. Whereas 75% of the patients had an open infarct-related artery documented at coronary angiography 2 hours after initiation of streptokinase infusion, only 45% showed recovery in regional function. Most of the patients showed recovery in function 3–10 days after therapy with only 1 showing recovery in function at 45 days. The best predictors of functional recovery were the presence of an open infarct-related artery (seen in all patients with functional recovery) and the duration between onset of symptoms and streptokinase therapy (those with functional recovery showing a shorter duration) [31].

Thus, although it is obvious that patients showing recovery in regional function have viable myocardium, does the lack of functional recovery denote the absence of viable myocardium? If we remember that the endocardium is responsible for most of the wall thickening, it is clear why some patients with open infarct-related arteries and viable myocardium do not show improvement in regional function; it is likely that in these patients the endocardium has been irreversibly damaged. Nevertheless, reperfusion therapy may have resulted in survival of the epicardial half of the myocardium. Whereas viable myocardium in the epicardial half may not cause recovery in regional function, it could prevent infarct expansion and left ventricular dilatation. Figure 6.9 illustrates the relation between the transmurality of infarction and infarct expansion. Less transmural infarcts, because they are surrounded by normal myocardium, will not expand and the left ventricle will not dilate (Figure 6.9A). In contrast, large infarcts, not having enough normal tissue to buttress them, will expand and

BASELINE   6 MONTHS LATER

A. SUBENDOCARDIAL INFARCTION

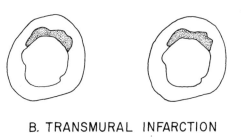

B. TRANSMURAL INFARCTION

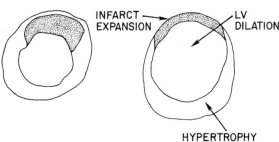

Figure 6.9. Relation between the transmurality of infarction and infarct expansion. Less transmural infarcts, because they are surrounded by normal myocardium, will not expand and the left ventricle will not dilate (A). In contrast, large infarcts, not having much normal tissue to buttress them, will expand and result in left ventricular dilatation (B).

result in left ventricular dilation (Figure 6.9). Thus, *the lack of infarct expansion is evidence for the presence* of viable myocardium.

In the study mentioned above where streptokinase was given within 4 hours of chest pain, most patients with open vessels who did not show functional recovery, failed to demonstrate infarct expansion and left ventricular dilation [31]. Only patients with closed vessels and large infarcts showed left ventricular dilation. In the GISSI study, patients who received streptokinase did not demonstrate an increase in left ventricular size between pre-discharge and 6-month follow-up studies compared to those who did not receive streptokinase; this latter group showed significant left ventricular enlargement 6 months after receiving the placebo [34].

Unlike the situation with the occluded infarct-related artery, where function has some relation to infarct size at the time of occlusion (Figure 6.3), in patients with open vessels, due to the post-ischemic state, myocardial function immediately after reperfusion is markedly depressed whether there is infarction or not and is not related to the size of the infarction. In these patients, dobutamine echocardiography has been used to determine the presence of viable myocardium [35–37]. The non-infarcted, post-ischemic myocardium, although dysfunctional, has contractile reserve [38–42] which can be elicited by catecholamine stimulation [39-42]. If the infarct-related artery is not flow-limiting, improvement in regional function will be seen with dobutamine when viable myocardium is present. If the lesion is flow-limiting, dobutamine may cause ischemia at higher doses which can result in deterioration of regional function. Since nonviable myocardium cannot be made ischemic, even worsening of function with dobutamine implies the presence of viable myocardium.

Does the degree of improvement in function during dobutamine infusion indicate the amount of viable myocardium and what is the dose of dobutamine needed to elicit contractile reserve? In an experimental study, coronary occlusion was performed for 2–6 hours to obtain infarcts of varying degrees of transmurality [43]. In half the dogs no dobutamine was given during any stage, while in the other half, 15 μg/kg/min of dobutamine was given at baseline, just before the release of the occlusion, and 15 minutes after release of the occlusion. In the group receiving no dobutamine, there was no relation between infarct size and wall thickening within the infarct bed either during coronary occlusion or 15 minutes after reperfusion (Figure 6.10A). In contrast, in those receiving dobutamine, while there was no relation between infarct size and wall thickening during coronary occlusion, a close inverse relation was noted between infarct size and wall thickening 15 minutes after reflow (Figure 6.10B): the less transmural the infarct (and hence, greater the amount of viable myocardium), the greater the degree of wall thickening in the presence of dobutamine. These results also suggest that while the epicardium does not contribute much to overall wall thickening at rest, its thickening is increased in the presence of dobutamine.

That the outer layers of the myocardium respond to inotropic stimulation has some interesting implications. Because of necrosis involving a critical extent of the myocardial thickness, as stated earlier, regional wall motion may be abolished at rest despite the presence of a significant amount of viable myocardium. During exercise or other forms of stress, however, where catecholamines are released, the outer layers of the myocardium may increase their thickening, thus enhancing wall motion and contributing to better overall left ventricular function. This kind of response might be important in preventing left ventricular dyssynergy and dilatation during stress and, hence, may contribute to improved functional status and survival in patients receiving successful thrombolysis even if they do not demonstrate spontaneous recovery in resting regional function.

In the experimental study referred to earlier [43], the dose of dobutamine required to elicit contractile reserve was related to the infarct size. If the infarct was small and located primarily within the inner one-fifth of the myocardium, 5 μg/kg/min of dobutamine was adequate to increase wall thickening. If the infarcts were larger, however, more dobutamine was needed. The ideal dose of dobutamine where a relation between infarct size and wall thickening could be established was 15 μg/kg/min. In these experiments, however, the infarct-related artery was not flow-limiting.

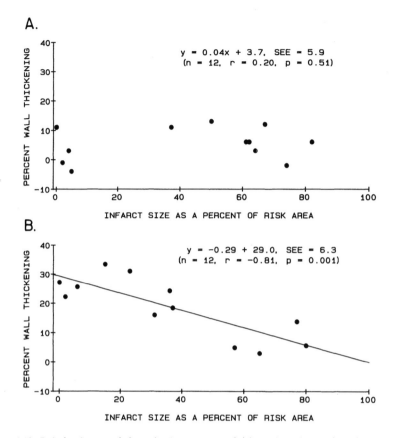

Figure 6.10. Relation between infarct size (as a percent of risk area) on the x-axis and percent wall thickening (on the y-axis) in the left anterior descending artery bed: A) after 2-4 hr of occlusion and 15 min of reflow in the absence of dobutamine, where no relation is noted between infarct size and percent wall thickening, and B) after 2–6 hr of occlusion and 15 min of reflow in the presence of 15 μ/kg/min of dobutamine, where an inverse linear relation is noted between infarct size and percent wall thickening: the larger the infarct, the less is the thickening, while more thickening is noted with smaller infarcts because of contractile reserve in the non-infarcted tissue that is unmasked in the presence of dobutamine. See text for details. From Sklenar *et al.* [43], with permission of the American Heart Association.

Clinical studies advocating 'low-dose' dobutamine (5 μg/kg/min) for detection of myocardial viability are different from this animal study in two major ways. First, the infarct-related artery may or may not be flow-limiting. In the former instance, higher doses of dobutamine may result in ischemia and worsening (rather than improvement) of wall motion. Second, these studies rely on ultimate spontaneous recovery in regional function as the hallmark of myocardial viability [35]. When spontaneous recovery in function occurs, only a small portion of the endocardium is infarcted and a 5 μg/kg/min dose is adequate to increase wall thickening. However, as stated earlier, a substantial portion of the myocardium can still be viable and now show spontaneous recovery in regional function. In such patients, a higher dose of dobutamine may be necessary to demonstrate an increase in wall thickening as long as the infarct-related artery is not flow-limiting.

Thus, using spontaneous recovery in regional function as the 'gold-standard' for myocardial viability may not be adequate in these kinds of patients, where dobutamine echocardiography, using a moderate dose of the drug, may better indicate the amount of viable myocardium. For instance, in a study using positron emission tomography, viability was noted in 11 of 17 patients with anterior myocardial infarction who had undergone successful thrombolysis within 3 hr of the onset of symptoms [37]. Although all 11 showed improvement in function with 10 μg/kg/min of dobutamine, only 6 showed spontaneous recovery later. Thus, dobutamine echocardiography at a moderate dose identified more viable myocardium than would have been predicted on the basis of spontaneous recovery in regional function.

Regional function in patients with chronic reduction in myocardial blood flow

Unfortunately, there is no animal model of chronic, persistent, hypoperfusion where flow-function relations can be studied. Models of short-term 'hibernation' have, however, been described [44]. It is not unreasonable to presume that the regional flow-function relation is somewhat like that noted during acute ischemia (Figure 6.2). In the clinical situation, severe narrowing of the epicardial coronary arteries is seen, which may also be occluded; in the latter situation, blood flow emanates from collaterals. The amount of flow in these situations is either not enough to sustain normal wall thickening (Figure 6.2) [44–46] or else basal flow is normal but repeated episodes of 'stunning' caused during periods of increased myocardial oxygen demand (such as exercise) are the basis of myocardial dysfunction [47].

Theoretically, the response of such myocardium to dobutamine could be unpredictable. If flow through the vessels can increase, then regional function should improve with dobutamine. On the other hand, if flow-limitation at rest is the major cause of myocardial dysfunction, function may either not improve with dobutamine (and may even worsen) or else may improve only briefly in response to catecholamine stimulation before getting worse [45]. In a recent study in patients with reduced global left ventricular function and multivessel disease, dobutamine echocardiography predicted improvement in function in those undergoing revascularization [48]. This prediction was based on improvement in function of dysfunctional segments at various doses of dobutamine. Two interesting findings of this study merit further investigation. One, it was not 'low-dose' dobutamine that resulted in improvement in function but, rather, the dose required to improve function varied anywhere from 5 μg/kg/min to 20 μg/kg/min, which where the minimal and maximal doses, respectively, used in the study. Second, patients with occluded vessels also demonstrated recovery in function which suggests that either collateral flow increased somewhat during the performance of the test to allow increase in wall thickening or the increase in wall thickening was based entirely on the chronotropic effects of dobutamine and was not associated with a concomitant increase in myocardial blood flow. The latter mechanism is more consistent with results from a similar experimental model [45]. In the model of acute coronary occlusion, interestingly, dobutamine does not enhance regional function [43]. Additional studies are needed to establish the role of dobutamine echocardiography in patients with hibernating myocardium.

Assessment of regional perfusion

Myocardial contrast echocardiography is a technique that utilizes the intravascular injection of microbubbles of air [49]. As these microbubbles traverse the myocardial microvasculature, they produce opacification of the myocardium on simultaneously performed echocardiography. These microbubbles remain entirely within the intravascular space and their presence within any myocardial region denotes the status of microvascular perfusion within that region [50, 51].

Contrast echocardiography during acute myocardial infarction when the infarct-related artery is occluded

In the absence of collateral blood flow, when a coronary artery is suddenly occluded, perfusion within the infarct zone is minimal and results in myocardial necrosis which starts in the endocardium and progresses transmurally over time (Figure 6.11) [21]. Within approximately 6 hours, the infarction is complete and any attempt at reperfusion after that is not beneficial. In fact, it may even be harmful since the infarct may become hemorrhagic with subsequent myocardial rupture. This principle forms the basis of early reperfusion in the setting of acute myocardial infarction, when early reflow arrests the transmural migration of infarction, resulting in myocardial salvage.

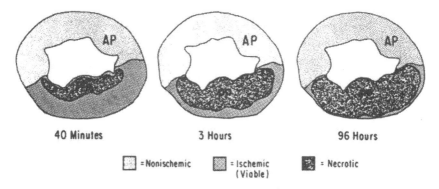

Figure 6.11. Relation between duration of coronary occlusion and infarct size as a percent of risk area. The infarct starts at the endocardium at 40 min into coronary occlusion and, in the absence of residual collateral-derived blood flow, migrates across the thickness of the myocardium in 6 hr. See text for details. From Reimer, Jennings [21], with permission.

In the presence of collateral-derived residual blood flow (as low as 0.2–0.3 ml/min/g), cell viability could be maintained within the occluded infarct bed [21]. At these low levels of flow, although regional function will be diminished (Figure 6.2), extensive necrosis may not occur and even late reperfusion may result in improvement in regional function. Heretofore, collateral vessels, like all coronary vessels, have been evaluated using coronary angiography. This technique, however, can only define vessels > 100 μ in diameter, while most collateral vessels are significantly smaller [52, 53]. Furthermore, the presence on angiography of a conduit connecting two epicardial vessels does not indicate whether the conduit is actually providing nutrient flow to myocardial cells.

Since it utilizes microbubbles with a mean size of 4–6 μ, myocardial contrast

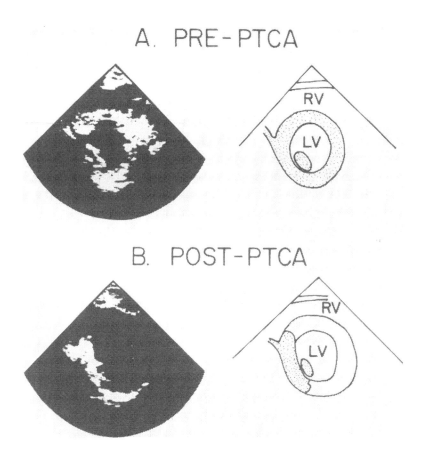

A. PRE-PTCA

B. POST-PTCA

Figure 6.12. Short-axis view of the left ventricle in a patient with an occluded right coronary artery. A) contrast was injected into the left main coronary artery prior to angioplasty of the right coronary artery. Homogeneous opacification of the entire myocardium, including the occluded right coronary artery bed is noted. B) contrast is injected selectively into the right coronary artery after successful angioplasty of that vessel. The latter injection defines the perfusion bed supplied by this artery which received collateral blood flow from the left coronary system when it was occluded (see A). From Sabia *et al.* [55], with permission.

echocardiography can be used to define the spatial distribution of residual collateral-derived blood flow within the infarct bed [54]. Figure 6.12 is an example of a patient with an inferior myocardial infarction and an occluded right coronary artery. When the bubbles were injected into the left main artery, not only did they opacify the left ventricular myocardium, but they also caused contrast enhancement of the occluded right coronary bed (Figure 6.12A), which implied that the right coronary bed received flow from the left coronary system through collateral vessels. The spatial extent of the right coronary bed in this patient was defined after opening the right coronary artery by angioplasty and injecting microbubbles directly into it (Figure 6.12B). It is evident that 100% of the right coronary bed received collateral flow from the left system in that particular short-axis view.

Another example is depicted in Figure 6.13 which illustrates the case of a

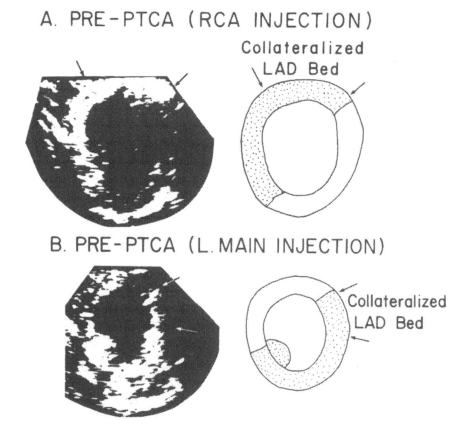

Figure 6.13. Illustrates end-diastolic frames from a patient with an occluded left anterior descending coronary artery after right (A) and left main coronary (B) injection of contrast. The regions subtended by arrows indicate the areas within the occluded bed supplied by collaterals from the right (A) and left circumflex (B) coronary arteries. See text for details. From Sabia *et al.* [54], with permission of the American Heart Association.

patient with an occluded left anterior descending artery. Injection of contrast into the right coronary artery not only resulted in opacification of the right coronary bed, but also of the medial portion of the left anterior descending bed (depicted by arrows in A). Similarly, on injecting contrast into the left main artery, not only was opacification noted in the left circumflex bed, but extended to the lateral portion of the occluded left anterior descending bed (depicted by arrows in B). This case, therefore, exemplifies the presence of both right-to-left and left-to-left collaterals which provide flow to nearly the entire left anterior descending bed in this short-axis view.

As would be expected, there is no correlation between angiographic collateral grade and the spatial extent of collateral perfusion defined by myocardial contrast echocardiography [54]. Patients with poor or no collaterals seen on angiography can have a large portion of the occluded bed supplied by collateral flow. It is also important to remember that collateral perfusion can be depicted on myocardial contrast echocardiography only when a gradient is present between one vessel and another. Thus, the bed to be studied should

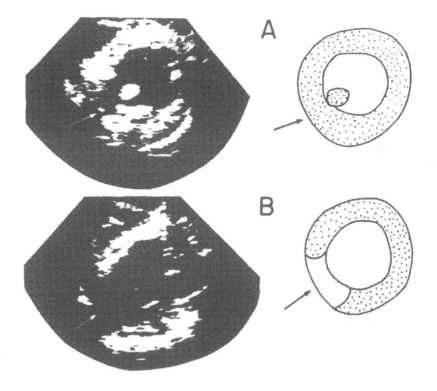

Figure 6.14. A) illustrates the second end-diastolic frame after left main injection of contrast in a patient with an occluded right coronary artery. Contrast appears at the same time in the occluded bed as in the normally perfused vessel. After successful angioplasty of the occluded right coronary artery, left main injection of contrast no longer results in opacification of the right coronary bed (B). See text for details. From Sabia *et al.* [54], with permission of the American Heart Association.

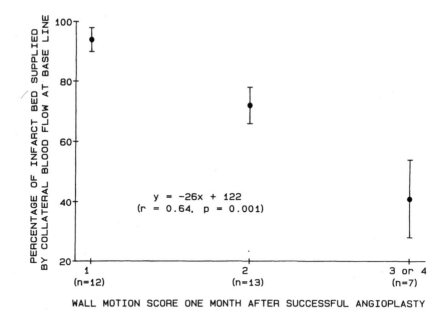

Figure 6.15. Correlation between wall motion score 1 month after successful angioplasty (where 1 = normal; 2 = mild hypokinesia; and, 3 and 4 are severe hypokinesia and akinesia, respectively) and percentage of the infarct bed supplied by collateral blood flow as defined by myocardial contrast echocardiography before angioplasty. From Sabia *et al.* [55], with permission.

either be totally or subtotally occluded. This is shown in Figure 6.14 using an example of a patient with inferior infarction. When contrast was injected into the left main artery in the presence of a totally occluded right coronary artery, collateral perfusion was noted in the right coronary bed (A). Immediately after opening the right coronary artery by angioplasty, however, injection of contrast in the left main artery could not opacify the right coronary bed (B). Thus, although collateral vessels were still present (since the two images were obtained only 1 hour apart), lack of a gradient between the left main and right coronary artery after angioplasty, failed to demonstrate their presence (B) [54].

The extent of the infarct bed supplied by collateral flow is a powerful predictor of improvement in function after successful angioplasty [55]. Figure 6.15 illustrates the relation between wall motion score 1 month after successful angioplasty and pre-angioplasty spatial extent of collateral perfusion in patients studies 2 days to 5 weeks after infarction, where lower wall motion scores indicate better function. Patients with extensive collateral perfusion of the infarct bed (> 50%) show marked improvement in function after successful angioplasty, while those with less extensive collateral perfusion do not show as good a recovery (Figure 6.16). Importantly, patients with good collateral flow who are not revascularized also do not demonstrate functional recovery. Furthermore, the time between infarction and angioplasty (up to 5 weeks in this study) does not influence these results. Thus, if adequate collateral-derived residual blood flow is present, it will maintain prolonged myocardial viability

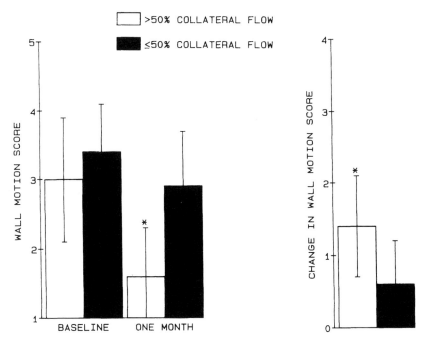

Figure 6.16. Comparison of mean wall motion scores in patients with good and poor collateral flow defined by myocardial contrast echocardiography. Good collateral flow was defined as > 50% of the infarct bed supplied by collateral flow, while poor collateral flow was defined as ≤ 50% of the bed supplied by collateral flow. Patients with good collateral flow showed significantly better function one month post-angioplasty compared to those with poor collateral flow (left, lower scores on the dependent axis represent better function, 1 = normal, 5 = dyskinesia). The improvement in wall motion score 1 month after angioplasty was also greater in those with good collateral blood flow (right). * indicates $P < 0.01$ (see text for details). From Sabia *et al.* [55].

and restoration of blood flow late after infarction will result in improvement in function [55].

Contrast echocardiography during acute myocardial infarction when the infarct-related artery is patent

In patients studied 1 day to 4 weeks after infarction, the extent of perfusion within the infarct bed defines recovery in function also in those who have open infarct-related arteries [56]. As depicted in Figure 6.17, if a segment has no perfusion it does not demonstrate improvement in function despite absence of a flow-limiting infarct-related artery. In contradistinction, segments within the same infarct bed showing adequate perfusion (Figure 6.17) exhibit improvement in function. Figure 6.18 illustrates the relation between the average perfusion score within an infarct bed and wall motion score 1 month later in patients with recent infarction who do not have flow-limiting infarct-related arteries. It is very likely that the regions showing perfusion with the artery open are the regions that have adequate collateral-derived perfusion during coronary occlusion and

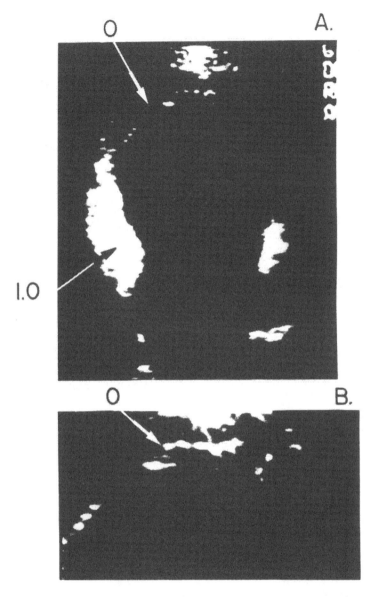

Figure 6.17. Example of perfusion patterns seen in a patient with an anteroapical infarction and an open infarct-related artery. While there was wall motion abnormality at baseline both in the apex and the interventricular septum, the former showed no opacification and the latter showed homogeneous opacification. After one month the apex did not show improvement in function while the interventricular septum exhibited significant improvement in function.

thus escape necrosis. Having escaped necrosis, both the myocardial cells and the microvasculature within these regions remain intact, while in regions that undergo necrosis (due to absence of adequate flow during occlusion), damage of

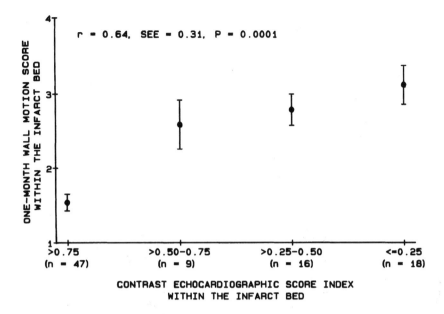

Figure 6.18. Correlation between one month wall motion score (scored as 1 = normal; 2 = mild hypokinesia; 3 = severe hypokinesia; 4 = akinesia; and, 5 = dyskinesia) on the *y*-axis, and the average contrast score within an infarct bed (each segment scored as 0 = no opacification; 0.5 = partial opacification; and, 1 = homogeneous opacification) on the *x*-axis, in 90 patients with recent infarction and an open infarct-related artery. See text for details. Adapted from Ragosta et al. [56], with permission of the American Heart Association.

the microvasculature is seen in conjunction with cellular death. It is for this reason that *microvascular perfusion is an indicator of cellular viability in patients examined later than 1 day after their infarction.*

Assessment of perfusion immediately after reperfusion is more complex for two major reasons. First, coronary hyperemia is noted for several hours after reperfusion, such that an indicator of microvascular perfusion (such as microbubbles) may underestimate the degree of necrosis [57–59]. Second, the perfusion pattern within the infarct bed undergoes dynamic changes in the first few hours after reperfusion, such that perfusion defects are more likely to be influenced as much by the timing of contrast injection as by the extent of microvascular injury [60, 61]. Despite hyperemia, however, the microvascular flow reserve within the infarct bed is abnormal and the region of abnormal flow reserve corresponds to the region of cellular necrosis [62–64]. Consequently, this abnormal physiology can be used to define regions with necrosis immediately after reflow despite coronary hyperemia and dynamic changes in the perfusion pattern that occur spontaneously within the infarct bed [65].

Figure 6.19 illustrates processed short-axis images in a dog who underwent 3 hours of reperfusion. Myocardial contrast echocardiography was performed at 45 minutes (A) and 3 hours into the reperfusion period before (B) and after (C) an intravenous infusion of dipyridamole. The echocardiographic images were processed using a method designed to optimally define gradations in contrast

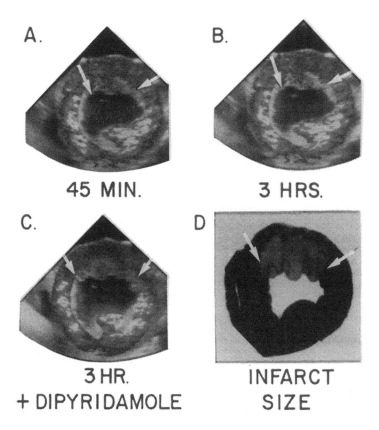

Figure 6.19. Changes in reperfusion patterns in a dog with a nearly transmural infarction. A) After 45 min of reperfusion, a small relative color defect localized to the endocardium in the anterior wall is noted as shown by arrows. B) After 3 hr of reperfusion, this defect was slightly larger as depicted by arrows. C) The addition of dipyridamole, resulted in a much larger relative contrast defect shown by arrows which closely delineated the true size and shape of the infarct on tissue staining with triphenyl tetrazolium chloride, which is indicated by arrows (D). See text for details. From Villanueva *et al.* [65], with permission of the American Heart Association.

enhancement, whereby gradations of red to orange, to yellow, to white, represented increasing degrees of contrast enhancement.

It can be appreciated from these illustrations that at 45 minutes into reflow (A), the anterior myocardium has less contrast effect (more red than yellow or white) compared to the posterior myocardium. However, the region with no color is located only within the endocardium and is slightly larger at 3 hours (B). After dipyridamole, however, the region with no color is much larger (C) and corresponds almost exactly with the infarct seen after triphenyl tetrazolium chloride staining of the heart (D). Thus, in the absence of dipyridamole, infarct size is underestimated both at 45 minutes and 3 hours after reflow. Microsphere data indicate that these findings are due to significant levels of flow to the infarct during the first few hours of reperfusion.

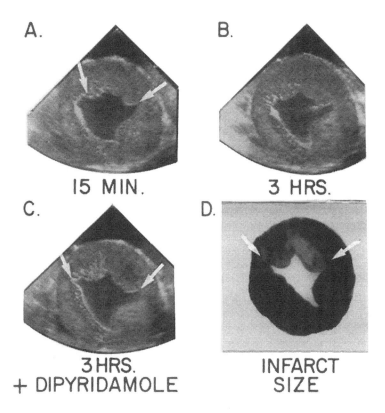

A. 15 MIN.

B. 3 HRS.

C. 3 HRS.
\+ DIPYRIDAMOLE

D. INFARCT
SIZE

Figure 6.20. Serial contrast defects in a dog with a moderate-sized infarct localized to the endocardial half of the anterior myocardium. A) After 15 min of reperfusion, a relative contrast defect involving almost the entire myocardial thickness of the anterior wall is noted as depicted by arrows. B) After 3 hr of reperfusion, almost no defect was seen. C) With the administration of dipyridamole at 3 hr, the region with no color indicated by arrows closely paralleled the size and distribution of the infarct delineated by triphenyl tetrazolium chloride staining (D). See text for details. From Villanueva *et al.* [65], with permission of the American Heart Association.

Another example is depicted in Figure 6.20 where myocardial contrast echocardiography performed 15 minutes after reflow shows a small endocardial perfusion defect in the anterior wall (A), while 3 hours after reflow, this defect has virtually disappeared (B). In the presence of dipyridamole, however, a butterfly-shaped defect is noted in the anterior wall (C) which corresponds very closely with the infarct size determined using triphenyl tetrazolium chloride (D). Thus, in the first few hours immediately after reperfusion, not only does myocardial contrast echocardiography underestimate infarct size in the absence of dipyridamole, but the perfusion defect size also changes dynamically.

Figure 6.21 illustrates the relation between perfusion defect and infarct size at 15 and 45 minutes and 2 and 3 hours after reperfusion. In each instance, there is marked underestimation of infarct size and only at 15 minutes after reperfusion a systemic relation is seen between perfusion bed and infarct size. In contradistinction, in the presence of dipyridamole, there is a close linear relation

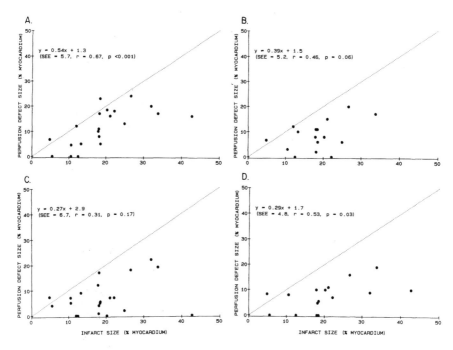

Figure 6.21. Relation between perfusion defect size defined on myocardial contrast echocardio-graphy (*y*-axis) and triphenyl tetrazolium-defined infarct size (*x*-axis) at A) 15 min, B) 45 min, C) 2 hr, and D) 3 hr after reflow. The dotted line in each panel depicts the line of identity. See text for details. From Villanueva *et al.* [65], with permission of the American Heart Association.

between perfusion defect and infarct size (Figure 6.22), with only a mild underestimation of infarct size by myocardial contrast echocardiography.

In the first few hours after reflow, therefore, it is only in the presence of a coronary vasodilator such as dipyridamole that perfusion defect size on myocardial contrast echocardiography corresponds to infarct size and the regions showing contrast uptake denote viable myocardium [66]. This phenomenon is observed because while immediately after reperfusion, flow to the infarct bed is increased, the flow reserve in this bed is abnormal. Thus, when dipyridamole is given, while flow to normal tissue increases several-fold above baseline, that to the infarct bed does not. When color-coding is used and white and yellow colors are assigned to the hyperemic normal beds, the infarct zone with impaired microvascular reserve is not assigned any color because *relative* to the posterior bed, flow there is very low.

Similar results have been demonstrated from left and right atrial injections of contrast in dogs [66]. Figure 6.23 illustrates an example of complete myocardial salvage after reperfusion in a dog in whom contrast was injected into the left atrium. A risk area is noted on contrast echocardiography during left anterior descending artery occlusion indicated by an anterior transmural relative color defect (A), which parallels the risk area on autoradiography (B). During reperfusion, contrast enhancement now occurs in this previously hypoperfused

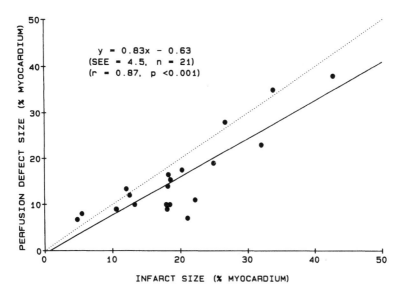

Figure 6.22. Relation between perfusion defect size defined on myocardial contrast echocardiography (*y*-axis) and triphenyl tetrazolium-defined infarct size (*x*-axis) after intravenous infusion of 0.56 mg/kg of dipyridamole. Unlike the situations in Figure 6.20, perfusion defect size is closely related to infarct size and only marginally underestimates it. See text for details. From Villanueva *et al.* [65], with permission of the American Heart Association.

area (C), indicated by oranges and yellows. The triphenyl tetrazolium chloride-stained slice shows no evidence of infarction (D). During these injections, although there is relative attenuation of the posterior segment of the heart due to left ventricular cavity opacification, the borders of the defect can nonetheless be seen.

Figure 6.24 exemplifies a nontransmural infarction in another dog receiving left atrial injection of contrast. Myocardial contrast echocardiography and technetium autoradiography concordantly show a transmural anterior defect (risk area) during left anterior descending artery occlusion (A and B, respectively). During reperfusion, the contrast defect persists, but it is no longer transmural (C). The subendocardial contrast defect corresponds to a nontransmural infarction indicated on the triphenyl tetrazolium chloride-stained slice (D). The subendocardial character of the contrast defect paralleled the reduced endocardial flow measured using radiolabeled microspheres. In both these examples (Figures 6.23 and 6.24), myocardial contrast echocardiography was performed in the presence of intravenous dipyridamole. Thus, while myocardial contrast echocardiography has been shown to define the 'no-reflow' phenomenon in patients in whom infarct artery patency has been established within a few hours of onset of chest pain [67], it is important to bear in mind that in the absence of a coronary vasodilator, the region with 'no flow' or 'low flow' will underestimate infarct size [68].

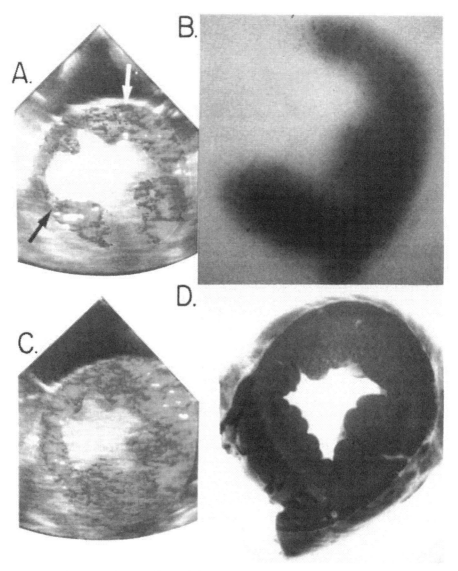

Figure 6.23. Example of successful reperfusion with no infarction and hence, complete myocardial salvage in a dog receiving left atrial injection of contrast. A) An anterior perfusion defect is noted on myocardial contrast echocardiography during left anterior descending coronary artery occlusion with B) a corresponding defect on technetium autoradiography. C) After reperfusion, there is no defect noted on myocardial contrast echocardiography and D) no infarction is noted on post-mortem triphenyl tetrazolium chloride staining of the heart. From Villanueva *et al.* [66], with permission of the American Heart Association.

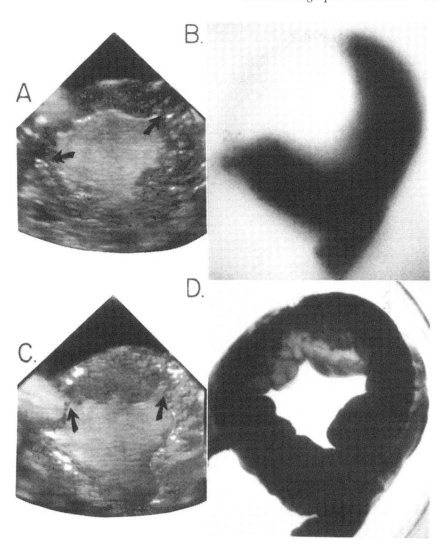

Figure 6.24. Example of successful reperfusion with partial myocardial salvage in a dog receiving left atrial injection of contrast. A) An anterior perfusion defect is noted on myocardial contrast echocardiography during left anterior descending coronary artery occlusion with B) a corresponding defect on technetium autoradiography. C) After reperfusion, an endocardial defect is noted on myocardial contrast echocardiography and D) a subendocardial infarction is noted on post-mortem triphenyl tetrazolium chloride staining of the heart. From Villanueva *et al.* [66], with permission of the American Heart Association.

Contrast echocardiography in patients with chronic reduction in myocardial blood flow

There are no published studies using contrast echocardiography in patients with multivessel disease and reduced global left ventricular function. Preliminary data from patients with moderately or severely reduced global left ventricular systolic function (left ventricular ejection fraction of $\leq$ 0.40) indicate that myocardial contrast echocardiography is useful for defining myocardial regions that will improve after revascularization [69]. Two issues need to be kept in mind in this group of patients. First, while improvement in function within a segment depends on the perfusion score of that segment, improvement in global left ventricular systolic function is influenced primarily by the number of segments showing contrast enhancement [69]. The more segments with contrast enhancement will result in better global left ventricular systolic function after revascularization. Second, successful revascularization of a segment is as essential a prerequisite for improvement in function as is the pattern of contrast enhancement. Technical problems during either angioplasty or bypass surgery, or poor distal runoff may preclude successful revascularization and thus, improvement in regional function despite contrast enhancement.

Summary

The flow-function relation may not only be different between individual patients, but also between individual segments within the same patient. These variations result from different pathophysiologic mechanisms of myocardial dysfunction within different myocardial segments in patients with coronary artery disease. Echocardiography offers a simple yet effective means of studying these relationships. For the reasons listed previously, it is the author's opinion that the response of the myocardium supplied by non flow-limiting lesions to dobutamine infusion should be used as the 'gold standard' for assessing presence of viable tissue rather than spontaneous recovery in regional function as is currently done. Additionally, lack of infarct expansion and left ventricular dilatation should also be considered as indicative of the presence of viable myocardium that is buttressing the infarct zone.

When perfusion and function information are used in the context of the clinical picture, myocardial contrast echocardiography can provide valuable information regarding the viability status of the myocardium in such patients. While the current applications of this technique are limited to intra-arterial injections performed in the cardiac catheterization laboratory [54–56, 67] and the operating room [70], with successful myocardial opacification from a venous injection [66, 71, 72], it has the potential for defining microvascular patency and hence myocardial viability in the outpatient laboratory.

References

1. Rahimtoola SH. A perspective on the three large multicenter randomized clinical trials of coronary bypass surgery for chronic stable angina. Circulation 1985; 72: V123-35.
2. Braunwald E, Kloner RA. The stunned myocardium: Prolonged, postischemic ventricular dysfunction. Circulation 1982; 66: 1146-9.
3. Brunken RC, Kottou S, Nienaber CA, Schwaiger M, Ratib OM, Phelps ME *et al.* PET detection of viable tissue in myocardial segments with persistent defects at Tl-201 SPECT. Radiology 1989; 172: 65-73.
4. Sabia PJ, Powers ER, Ragosta M, Smith WH, Watson DD, Kaul S. Role of quantitative planar thallium-201 imaging for determining viability in patients with acute myocardial infarction and a totally occluded infarct-related artery. J Nucl Med 1993; 34: 728-36.
5. Ragosta M, Beller GA, Watson DD, Kaul S, Gimple LW. Quantitative planar rest-redistribution ^{201}Tl imaging in detection of myocardial viability and prediction of improvement in left ventricular function after coronary bypass surgery in patients with severely depressed left ventricular function. Circulation 1993; 87: 1630-41.
6. Sinusas AJ, Trautman KA, Bergin JD, Watson DD, Ruis M, Smith WH *et al.* Quantification of area at risk during coronary occlusion and degree of myocardial salvage after reperfusion with technetium-99m methoxyisobutyl isonitrile. Circulation 1990; 82: 1424-37.
7. Kaul S. Echocardiography in coronary artery disease. Curr Probl Cardiol 1990; 15: 233-98.
8. Myers JH, Stirling MC, Choy M, Buda AJ, Gallagher KP. Direct measurement of inner and outer wall thickening dynamics with epicardial echocardiography. Circulation 1986; 74: 164-72.
9. Weintraub WS, Hattori S, Aggarwal JB, Bodenheimer MM, Banks VS, Helfant RH. The relationship between myocardial blood flow and contraction by myocardial layer in the canine left ventricle during ischemia. Circ Res 1981; 48: 430-8.
10. Gallagher KP, Matsuzaki M, Koziol JA, Kemper WS, Ross J Jr. Regional myocardial perfusion and wall thickening during ischemia in conscious dogs. Am J Physiol 1984; 247: H727-38.
11. Vatner SF. Correlation between acute reductions in myocardial blood flow and function in conscious dogs. Circ Res 1980; 47: 201-7.
12. Meyer SL, Curry GC, Donsky MS, Twieg DB, Parkey RW, Willerson JT. Influence of dobutamine on hemodynamic and coronary blood flow in patients with and without coronary artery disease. Am J Cardiol 1976; 38: 103-8.
13. Ricci DR, Orlick AE, Alderman EL, Ingels NB Jr, Daughters GT 2d, Kusnick CA *et al.* Role of tachycardia as inotropic stimulus in man. J Clin Invest 1979; 63: 695-703.
14. Sonnenblick EH, Frishman WH, LeJemtel TH. Dobutamine: A new synthetic cardioactive sympathetic amine. N Engl J Med 1979; 300: 17-22.
15. Gregg DE. Effect of coronary perfusion pressure or coronary flow on oxygen usage of the myocardium. Circ Res 1986; 13: 497-500.
16. Liberman AN, Weiss JL, Judgutt BI, Becker LC, Bulkley BH, Garrison JG *et al.* Two-dimensional echocardiography and infarct size: Relationship of regional wall motion and thickening to the extent of myocardial infarction in the dog. Circulation 1981; 63: 739-46.
17. Kaul S, Pandian NG, Gillam LD, Newell JB, Okada RD, Weyman AE. Contrast echocardiography in acute myocardial ischemia. III. An *in vivo* comparison of the extent of abnormal wall motion with the area at risk for necrosis. J Am Coll Cardiol 1986; 7: 383-92.
18. Wyatt HL, Da Luz PL, Waters DD, Swan HJ, Forrester JS. Contrasting influences of alterations in ventricular preload and afterload upon systemic hemodynamics, function, and metabolism in ischemic myocardium. Circulation 1977; 55: 318-24.
19. Sklenar J, Jayaweera AR, Kaul S. A computer-aided approach for the quantitation of left ventricular function using two-dimensional echocardiography. J Am Soc Echocardiogr 1992; 5: 33-40.
20. Gibbons EF, Hogan FD, Franklin TD, Nolting M, Weyman AE. The natural history of regional dysfunction in a canine preparation of chronic infarction. Circulation 1985; 71: 394-402.

21. Reimer KA, Jennings RB. The 'wavefront phenomenon' of myocardial ischemic cell death. II. Transmural progression of necrosis within the framework of ischemic bed size (myocardium at risk) and collateral flow. Lab Invest 1979; 40: 633–44.

22. Ross J Jr. Assessment of ischemic regional myocardial dysfunction and its reversibility. Circulation 1986; 74: 1186–90.

23. Matsuzaki M, Gallagher KP, Kemper WS, White F, Ross J Jr. Sustained regional dysfunction produced by prolonged coronary stenosis: Gradual recovery after reperfusion. Circulation 1983; 68: 170–82.

24. Robertson WS, Feigenbaum H, Armstrong WH, Dillon JC, O'Donnell J, McHenry PW. Exercise echocardiography: A clinically practical addition in the evaluation of coronary artery disease. J Am Coll Cardiol 1983; 2: 1085–91.

25. Homans DC, Sublett E, Dai XZ, Bache RJ. Persistence of regional left ventricular dysfunction after exercise-induced myocardial ischemia. J Clin Invest 1986; 77: 66–73.

26. Kloner RA, Allen J, Cox TA, Zheng Y, Ruiz CE. Stunned left ventricular myocardium after exercise treadmill testing in coronary artery disease. Am J Cardiol 1991; 68: 329–34.

27. Nixon JV, Brown CN, Smitherman TC. Identification of transient and persistent segmental wall motion abnormalities in patients with unstable angina by two-dimensional echocardiography. Circulation 1982; 65: 1497–503.

28. Marzullo P, Parodi O, Sambuceti G, Marcassa C, Gimelli A, Bartoli M et al. Does the myocardium become 'stunned' after episodes of angina at rest, angina on effort, and coronary angioplasty? Am J Cardiol 1993; 71: 1045–51.

29. Charuzi Y, Beeder C, Marshall LA, Sasaki H, Pack NB, Geft I et al. Improvement in regional and global left ventricular function after intracoronary thrombolysis: Assessment with two-dimensional echocardiography. Am J Cardiol 1984; 53: 662–5.

30. Widemsky P, Cervenka V, Gregor P, Visek V, Slakova T, Dvorak J et al. First month course of left ventricular asynergy after intracoronary thrombolysis in acute myocardial infarction. A longitudinal echocardiographic study. Eur Heart J 1985; 6: 759–65.

31. Touchstone DA, Beller GA, Nygaard TW, Tedesco C, Kaul S. Effects of successful intravenous reperfusion therapy on regional myocardial function and geometry in man: A tomographic assessment using two-dimensional echocardiography. J Am Coll Cardiol 1989; 13: 1506–13.

32. Oh JK, Gersh BJ, Nassef LA Jr, Miller FA Jr, Chesebro JH, Holmes DR Jr et al. Effects of acute reperfusion on regional myocardial function: Serial two-dimensional echocardiography assessment. Int J Cardiol 1989; 22: 161–8.

33. Penco M, Romano S, Agati L, Dagianti A, Vitavelli A, Fedele F et al. Influence of reperfusion induced by thrombolytic treatment on natural history of left ventricular regional motion abnormality in acute myocardial infarction. Am J Cardiol 1993; 71: 1015–20.

34. Marino P, Zanolla L, Zardini P. Effect of streptokinase on left ventricular modeling and function after myocardial infarction: The GISSI (gruppo Italiano per lo Studio della Streptochinasi nell'Infarto Miocardico) Trial. J Am Coll Cardiol 1989; 14: 1149–58.

35. Smart SC, Sawada SC, Ryan T, Segar D, Atherton L, Berkovitz K et al. Low-dose dobutamine echocardiography detects reversible dysfunction after thrombolytic therapy of acute myocardial infarction. Circulation 1993; 88: 405–15.

36. Barilla F, Cheorghiade M, Alam M, Khaja F, Goldstein S. Low-dose dobutamine in patients with acute myocardial infarction identifies viable but not contractile myocardium and predicts the magnitude of improvement in wall motion abnormalities in response to coronary revascularization. Am Heart J 1991; 122: 1522–31.

37. Pierard LA, De Landsheere CM, Berthe C, Rigo P, Kulbertus HE. Identification of viable myocardium by echocardiography during dobutamine infusion in patients with myocardial infarction after thrombolytic therapy: comparison with position emission tomography. J Am Coll Cardiol 1990; 15: 1021–31.

38. Stahl LD, Aversano TR, Becker LC. Selective enhancement of function of stunned myocardium by increased flow. Circulation 1986; 74: 843–51.

39. Becker LC, Levine JH, DiPaula AF, Guarnieri T, Aversano T. Reversal of dysfunction in

postischemic stunned myocardium by epinephrine and postextrasystolic potentiation. J Am Coll Cardiol 1986; 7: 580-9.

40. Bolli R, Zhu W, Myers MR, Hartley CJ, Roberts R. Beta-adrenergic stimulation reverses postischemic myocardial dysfunction without producing subsequent functional deterioration. Am J Cardiol 1985; 56: 964-8.

41. Mercier JC, Lando U, Kanmatsuse K, Ninomiya K, Meerbaum S, Fishbein MC *et al.* Divergent effects of inotropic stimulation on the ischemic and severely depressed reperfused myocardium. Circulation 1982; 66: 397-400.

42. Ellis SG, Wynne J, Braunwald E, Henschke CI, Sandor T, Kloner RA. Response of reperfusion-salvaged, stunned myocardium to inotropic stimulation. Am Heart J 1984; 107: 13-9.

43. Sklenar J, Villanueva FS, Glasheen WP, Ismail S, Goodman NC, Kaul S. Dobutamine echocardiography for determining the extent of myocardial salvage after reperfusion: An experimental evaluation. Circulation; In press.

44. Schulz R, Guth BD, Pieper K, Martin C, Heusch G. Recruitment of an inotropic reserve in moderately ischemic myocardium at the expense of metabolic recovery: A model of short-term hibernation. Circ Res 1992; 70: 1282-95.

45. Schulz R, Rose J, Martin C, Brodde OE, Heusch G. Development of short-term myocardial hibernation. Its limitation by the severity of ischemia and inotropic stimulation. Circulation 1993; 88: 684-95.

46. Parodi O, Maria RD, Oltrona L, Testa R, Sambuceti G, Roghi A *et al.* Myocardial blood flow distribution in patients with ischemic heart disease or dilated cardiomyopathy undergoing heart transplantation. Circulation 1993; 88: 509-22.

47. Vanoverschelde JL, Wijns W, Depre C, Essamri B, Heyndrickx GR, Borgers M *et al.* Mechanisms of chronic regional postischemic dysfunction in humans. New insights from the study of noninfarcted collateral-dependent myocardium. Circulation 1993; 87: 1513-23.

48. Cigarroa CG, deFillipi CR, Brickner E, Alvarez LG, Wait MA, Grayburn PA. Dobutamine stress echocardiography identifies hibernating myocardium and predicts recovery of left ventricular function after coronary revascularization. Circulation 1993; 88: 430-6.

49. Kaul S, Force T. Assessment of myocardial perfusion with contrast two-dimensional echocardiography. In Weyman AE (ed): Principles and Practice of Echocardiography. 2nd ed. Philadelphia: Lea and Febiger 1993: 687-720.

50. Kaul S. Clinical applications of myocardial contrast echocardiography. Am J Cardiol 1992; 69: 46H-55H.

51. Kaul S, Jayaweera AR. Myocardial contrast echocardiography has the potential for the assessment of coronary microvascular reserve. J Am Coll Cardiol 1993; 21: 356-8.

52. Cohen MV. Coronary collaterals: Clinical and Experimental Observations. Mount Kisco, NY: Futura 1985: 1-91.

53. Gensini GG, Bruto daCosta BC. The coronary collateral circulation in living man. Am J Cardiol 1969; 24: 393-400.

54. Sabia PJ, Powers ER, Jayaweera AR, Ragosta M, Kaul S. Functional significance of collateral blood flow in patients with recent acute myocardial infarction. A study using myocardial contrast echocardiography. Circulation 1992; 85: 2080-9.

55. Sabia PJ, Powers ER, Ragosta M, Saremblock IJ, Burwell LR, Kaul S. An association between collateral blood flow and myocardial viability in patients with recent myocardial infarction. N Engl J Med 1992; 372: 1825-31.

56. Ragosta M, Camarano G, Kaul S, Powers ER, Sarembock IJ, Gimple LW. Microvascular Integrity indicates myocellular viability in patients with recent myocardial infarction: New insights using myocardial contrast echocardiography. Circulation 1994; 89: 2562-9.

57. White FC, Sanders M, Bloor CM. Regional redistribution of myocardial blood flow after coronary occlusion and reperfusion in the conscious dog. Am J Cardiol 1978; 42: 234-43.

58. Heyndrickx GR, Amano J, Patrick TA, Manders WT, Rogers GG, Rosendorff C *et al.* Effects of coronary artery reperfusion on regional myocardial blood flow and function in conscious baboons. Circulation 1985; 71: 1029-37.

59. Cobb FR, Bache RJ, Rivas F, Greenfield JC Jr. Local effects of acute cellular injury on regional myocardial blood flow. J Clin Invest 1976; 57: 1359–68.
60. Ambrosio G, Weisman HF, Mannisi JA, Becker LC. Progressive impairment of regional myocardial perfusion after initial restoration of postischemic blood flow. Circulation 1989; 80: 1846–61.
61. Knabb RM, Bergmann SR, Fox KA, Sobel BE. The temporal pattern of recovery of myocardial perfusion and metabolic delineated by positron emission tomography after coronary thrombolysis. J Nucl Med 1987; 28: 1563–70.
62. Kloner RA, Ellis SG, Lange R, Braunwald E. Studies of experimental coronary artery reperfusion. Effects on infarct size, myocardial function, biochemistry, ultrastructure and microvascular damage. Circulation 1983; 68: I8–15.
63. Johnson WB, Malone SA, Pantely GA, Anselone CG, Bristow JD. No reflow and extent of infarction during maximal vasodilation in the porcine heart. Circulation 1988; 78: 462–72.
64. Vanhaecke J, Flameng W, Borgers M, Jang IK, Van de Werf F, De Geest H. Evidence for decreased coronary flow reserve in viable postischemic myocardium. Circ Res 1990; 67: 1201–10.
65. Villanueva FS, Glasheen WP, Sklenar J, Kaul S. Characterization of spatial patterns of flow within the reperfused myocardium using myocardial contrast echocardiography. Implications in determining the extent of myocardial salvage. Circulation 1993; 88: 2596–606.
66. Villanueva FS, Glasheen WP, Sklenar J, Kaul S. Assessment of risk area during coronary occlusion and infarct size after reperfusion with myocardial contrast echocardiography using left and right atrial injections of contrast. Circulation 1993; 88: 596–604.
67. Ito H, Tomooka T, Sakai N, Yu H, Higashino Y, Fujii K *et al.* Lack of myocardial perfusion immediately after successful thrombolysis. A predictor of poor recovery of left ventricular function in anterior myocardial infarction. Circulation 1992; 85: 1699–705.
68. Kaul S, Villanueva FS. Is the determination of myocardial perfusion necessary to evaluate the success of reperfusion when the infarct-related artery is open? Circulation 1992; 85: 1942–4.
69. Camarano GP, Ragosta M, Gimple LW, Powers E, Kaul S. Identification of viable myocardium with contrast echo in patients with myocardial infarction and poor left ventricular function. J Am Coll Cardiol 1994; 23: 450A (Abstract).
70. Spotnitz WD, Kaul S. Intraoperative assessment of myocardial perfusion using contrast echocardiography. Echocardiography 1990; 7: 209–28.
71. Villanueva FS, Glasheen WP, Sklenar J, Jayaweera AR, Kaul S. Successful and reproducible myocardial opacification during two-dimensional echocardiography from right heart injection of contrast. Circulation 1992; 85: 1557–64.
72. Ismail S, Jayaweera AR, Camarano G, Goodman NC, Skyba DD, Kaul S. Coronary stenosis can be detected by myocardial contrast echocardiography using left and right atrial injection of contrast. Circulation 1993; 88 (Suppl. I): I-303 (Abstract).

7. Magnetic resonance techniques for the assessment of myocardial viability

ERNST E. VAN DER WALL & HUBERT W. VLIEGEN

Introduction

With the application of magnetic resonance (MR) imaging techniques in clinical cardiology, important tools have been added to the currently available diagnostic arsenal for the evaluation of patients with coronary artery disease [1,2].

In patients with coronary artery disease, it is of paramount importance to distinguish ischemic but viable myocardium from areas of myocardial fibrosis. Viable myocardial areas are most likely to benefit from revascularization, whereas revascularization of fibrotic myocardium will not lead to improvement of left ventricular function.

Perfusion disturbances lead to myocardial ischemia, resulting in stunning, hibernation or necrosis. Myocardial stunning is a reversible state of reduced contractility, occurring directly following myocardial ischemia. Hibernation is a prolonged subacute or chronic stage of myocardial ischemia without pain, but with reduced myocardial contractility [3]. Hibernating myocardium is viable, jeopardized myocardium that shows improvement of contractility and left ventricular function after adequate blood supply is restored [4,5]. Persistent, dysfunctional, nonviable myocardium results from completed infarction (necrosis). Accordingly, definitive evidence of myocardial viability is the temporal improvement in contractile function, irrespective of the etiology of the dysfunction or the specific therapeutic intervention employed [6,7]. For the prospective identification of jeopardized but viable myocardium for purposes of guiding therapeutic interventions in individual patients, the following three standards for myocardial viability can be used:

1. preserved coronary flow (adequate perfusion)
2. preserved wall motion (systolic wall thickening)
3. preserved metabolism (presence of metabolic integrity)

The current MR techniques provide great potential to measure all three standards of viability [8,9]. Adequate perfusion can be assessed by *spin-echo MR imaging* or *ultrafast MR imaging*, systolic wall thickening by *cine MR imaging*, and the presence of metabolic integrity can be determined by *MR spectroscopy*.

In this chapter, an overview will be given of the assessment of viability using the various MR techniques. These non-invasive and versatile techniques have

A.S. Iskandrian and E.E. van der Wall (eds): Myocardial viability, 103–140.
© 1994 *Kluwer Academic Publishers.*

led toward increasing interest and research in the past few years. Particular strengths of the MR techniques are:

1. the inherent three-dimensional data acquisition without radiation exposure
2. the intrinsic soft tissue contrast which allows tissue characterization
3. the excellent spatial resolution (in the 1–2 mm range) which permits the evaluation of regional abnormalities
4. multitomographic imaging capabilities which allow acquisition of cardiac images in any plane
5. the inherent sensitivity to blood and wall motion
6. the potential of *in vivo* measurement of myocardial biochemistry using MR spectroscopy

To date, the majority of research has been focused on detection of myocardial perfusion abnormalities and on cardiac wall motion studies. Few clinical studies have been performed on cardiac metabolism using spectroscopy but the information gained is unique, necessitating further exploration of this modality in the assessment of cardiac metabolism and viability.

Coronary perfusion

Myocardial tissue characterization using MR imaging

MR imaging is well suited for the evaluation of myocardial ischemia and infarction using its capabilities of tissue characterization. Myocardial ischemia and infarction are associated with increased myocardial signals as a result of prolonged tissue relaxation times T1 and T2 (T1 = longitudinal relaxation time and T2 = transverse relaxation time) [10,11]. The increase in relaxation times results in changes in image intensity. The magnitude of increase in T1 and T2 is proportional to the magnitude of changes in blood flow. Changes in T1 and T2 can be detected *in vivo* from 3 to 6 hours after coronary artery occlusion and may persist for 20 days [12].

Experimental studies

MR imaging of dogs with reperfused myocardium have shown a significant increase in signal intensity and T2 relaxation times as early as 30 minutes after reperfusion [13–19]. These studies indicated that MR imaging detects ischemic myocardial areas soon after coronary occlusion, thereby providing a method to discern reperfused viable myocardium. MR imaging allows the assessment of infarct size based on different T2-relaxation times between infarcted and normal tissue [20,21]. However, infarct size may be slightly overestimated, particularly in the case of smaller, nontransmural infarctions [22]. In fact, the best correlation is found between MR infarct size and the hypoperfused myocardium, i.e. the region with a greater than 25% reduction of flow compared with control. Serial MR studies in dogs after varying times of occlusion, either with or without reperfusion, showed that T1 and T2 abnormalities did not correlate very well with the infarct zone prior to three weeks after occlusion, implying that MR imaging may not be suitable for early detection of infarct size [23]. On the other hand, serial MR imaging of left ventricular infarct size 3 and 21 days after coronary artery ligation using T2 measurements correlated well with histopathologically assessed infarct size [24]. Based on these experimental findings, a T2 strategy has been advocated to evaluate healing patterns in patients following reperfusion after thrombolytic therapy [25]. Therefore, MR imaging may identify both viable and nonviable myocardium due to its tissue characterization capabilities.

Clinical studies

Clinical studies in patients with documented myocardial infarction have also shown T1 and T2 alterations in infarcted myocardium. McNamara *et al.* [26] studied nine patients with acute myocardial infarction 5 to 12 days after the acute onset and showed that the infarcted areas were characterized by increased signal intensity of the infarcted region and prolonged T2 relaxation time. Distinction between normal and infarcted myocardium was sufficient to estimate infarct size. Johnston *et al.* [27] studied 34 patients 3 to 30 days after myocardial infarction, and showed that regional increase of signal intensity was consistent with the electrocardiographic location of the infarction and with the presence of hypokinetic segments on the left ventriculogram. Fisher *et al.* [28] showed in 29 patients, 3 to 17 days after myocardial infarction, prolonged T2 relaxation times in infarcted myocardial regions. On the other hand, they observed that increased signal intensity on T2-weighted images may be very difficult to distinguish from slowly moving intraventricular blood flow. In addition, Ahmad *et al.* [29] showed that T2 prolongation might not be a specific marker for acute myocardial infarction, as it can also be observed in abnormally perfused myocardial segments of patients with unstable angina. Been *et al.* [30] demonstrated in 10 of 13 patients with recent myocardial infarction a 40% increase of T1 values in the infarcted areas. In a subsequent study, Been *et al.* [31] showed in 41 patients with acute myocardial infarction that maximum T1 values were observed 2 weeks after the acute onset, suggesting that the increase of T1 reflects cellular infiltration as much as, or more than, tissue edema. No differences in T1 values were observed between the patients with or without reperfusion, indicating that alterations of T1 are complex and may bear no relationship with specific histological findings.

In the absence of any histologic confirmation, these statements remain purely speculative. Studies from our institution by Postema *et al.* [32] and Krauss *et al.* [33] showed that regional T2-abnormalities in 82% of 20 patients with acute myocardial infarction, who underwent MR studies with a mean of 8 days after the acute event, correlated with the presence and location of thallium-201 perfusion defects at rest. These studies emphasized the value of MR tissue

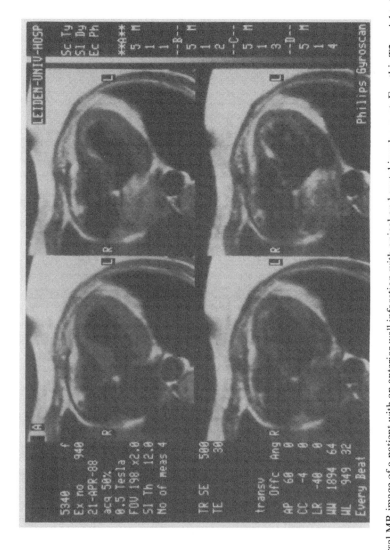

Figure 7.1. Transversal MR image of a patient with an anterior wall infarction with apical and septal involvement. For this T2-weighted MR image a multi-echo study (TE 30-60-90-120 msec) was performed. Note the increased signal intensity of the antero-apical wall on the even echo's (TE 60-120 msec, images on the right side). Also wall thinning and dilatation of the left ventricle is noticed at the apical and septal wall.

characterization in flow-deprived, injured myocardial tissue. Krauss *et al.* [34] showed in patients 7 to 14 days after acute myocardial infarction that MR imaging provided an accurate means of assessing infarct size, based on the calculation of T2 relaxation times. An example of an MR image obtained in a patient with a recent myocardial infarction is shown in Figure 7.1. In a subsequent study, good agreements were found between enzymatic infarct size, thallium-201 scintigraphy, radionuclide angiography and MR findings [35].

In addition to changes in T1 and T2 relaxation times as indices for tissue characterization, other characteristics can also be used to indicate infarcted myocardial areas, such as increased signal intensity, ventricular cavitary signal and regional wall thinning. Filipchuk *et al.* [36] showed increased myocardial signal intensity in 88%, cavitary signal in 74%, and regional wall thinning in 67% of 27 patients with acute myocardial infarction. However, in 18 asymptomatic volunteers increased myocardial signal intensity was also observed in 83%, cavitary signal in 94%, and wall thinning in 11% of cases. These findings imply that increased signals, both from myocardial tissue and the cavity, are sensitive but not at all specific for myocardial infarction. Of the three features, therefore, wall thinning was the most predictive and specific for acute myocardial infarction (Figure 7.2). In 17 patients with a recent myocardial infarction, White *et al.* [37] showed a high correlation between MR imaging and two-dimensional echocardiography for demonstrating regional wall motion abnormalities. They extended this study to 22 patients and observed that the extent of regional wall thinning by MR imaging can be used to measure infarct size [38]. Wisenberg *et al.* [39] showed in 66 patients 3 weeks after acute infarction that infarct size could very well be determined by MR imaging based on signal intensity. They demonstrated that, in the 41 patients who had received acute streptokinase therapy, a significant reduction in MR-measured infarct size was observed, compared to the patients without thrombolytic therapy. Johns *et al.* [40] assessed MR infarct size in 20 patients based on signal intensity at a mean of 9 days after the acute onset of symptoms. MR infarct size correlated very well with the extent of the region with severe hypokinesia visualized by left ventricular angiography. Turnbull *et al.* [41] compared MR imaging, based on T1 maps, with enzymatic infarct size, technetium-99m pyrophosphate scintigraphy, and radionuclide angiography in 19 patients 5 to 7 days following myocardial infarction. The authors found a strong agreement between infarct size detected by MR imaging and that assessed by the radionuclide techniques.

In summary, myocardial ischemia is associated with prolonged T1 and T2 relaxation times. Using T2-weighted images, a region with increased signal intensity can be delineated. However, regions with increased signal intensity may indicate either myocardial infarction or hypoperfused myocardium. Therefore, the use of signal intensities alone may not be specific enough to distinguish viable from nonviable myocardium. Additional morphological MR features are useful, such as increased intracavitary signal and regional wall thinning, to distinguish nonviable infarcted tissue from viable hypoperfused

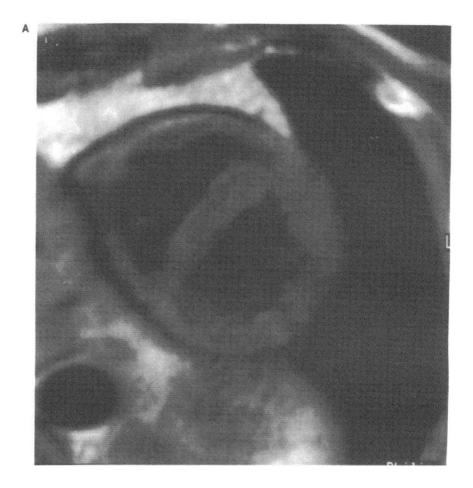

Figure 7.2A. Cardiac short-axis MR image of patient without cardiac disease. Myocardial walls of left and right ventricle are clearly depicted.

tissue. The accurate determination of infarct size by spin-echo MR imaging may prove useful in assessing new treatments designed to salvage myocardium.

Contrast agents

The identification of ischemic and infarcted tissue by MR imaging has been greatly improved by the use of paramagnetic contrast agents [42]. Despite the ability to generate images with varying image contrast, using the relaxation parameters T1 and T2, it is far from easy to detect abnormalities in tissue physiology in the early stage of myocardial ischemia without paramagnetic contrast agents. Besides, the detection of acute infarction with unenhanced MR imaging does not occur until several hours after coronary occlusion. Therefore, paramagnetic contrast agents have been developed to define functional and

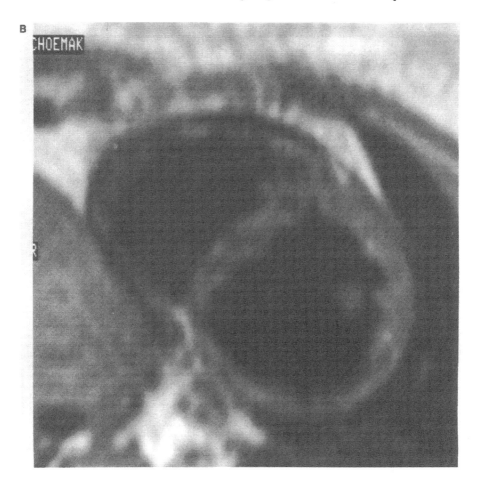

Figure 7.2B. Short-axis MR image of a patient with a two-week old myocardial infarction of the inferoposterior wall. There is marked wall thinning of the inferoposterior wall and a clear dilatation of the left ventricle.

perfusion abnormalities in the setting of acute myocardial ischemia and infarction [43–53].

Paramagnetic compounds cause a shortening of both the T1 and T2 relaxation times with the T1 relaxation time predominating. The magnitude of the change in relaxation time is influenced by both magnetic field strength and agent concentration. Local tissue perfusion is thus delineated in a manner analogous to standard indicator dilution methods, with more pronounced effects seen in areas of highest contrast agent concentration. In particular, gadolinium-containing contrast agents (labeled with DTPA, DOTA or albumin) have been shown to provide contrast on MR images. Most clinical experience has been obtained with Gadolinium (Gd)-DTPA, which can be safely used in patients with coronary artery disease and provides a better image quality than T2-weighted images [54].

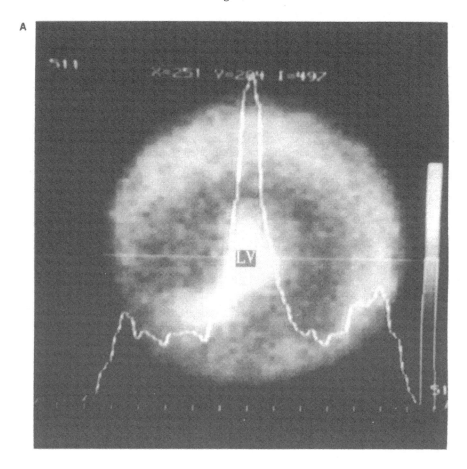

Figure 7.3A. Magnetic resonance image of midventricular slice of an isolated rat heart with 120 minutes of ischemia (no reperfusion; end-ischemic coronary flow, 19% of the pre-ischemic value). After 5 minutes of Gd-DTPA washing, a sharply delineated transition zone between areas with high and low signal intensity is visible. The intensity scan is recorded along a line drawn across the image.

Experimental studies with Gd-DTPA

Gd-DTPA has been shown to improve contrast enhancement of ischemic and infarcted myocardium in dogs [55–59]. Both T1 and T2 relaxation times are significantly shortened by Gd-DTPA in ischemic myocardial tissue after experimental coronary artery occlusion. The effect on T1 relaxation time is predominant and therefore T1-weighted images are used. These images show enhanced signal intensity in ischemic myocardium after administration of Gd-DTPA. The contrast enhancement at the ischemic area is probably caused by differences in wash-in and wash-out of Gd-DTPA from normal and ischemic myocardium. In acutely damaged myocardium, the increased accumulation of Gd-DTPA is dependent on blood flow, tissue blood volume, the size of the

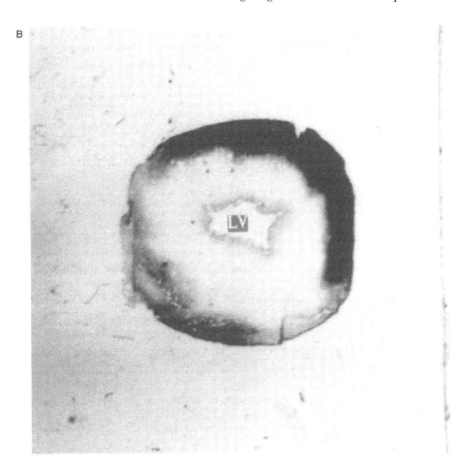

Figure 7.3B. Evans blue image of a midventricular slice of a heart with 120 minutes of ischemia (no reperfusion; end-ischemic coronary flow, 21% of the pre-ischemic value). A large area extending from subendocardial to mesocardial layers is free of Evans blue stain. LV = left ventricular cavity. (Reproduced with permission, from Holman *et al.* [66].)

extracellular space, and the permeability of the capillaries, all of which causes slow wash-out from the infarcted zone. Gd-DTPA is largely washed out of the normal myocardium 10 to 15 minutes after injection, while it remains in the infarcted zone. This suggests that MR imaging is preferably performed *after* 15 to 25 minutes. Gd-DTPA remains extracellular and is excreted by glomerular filtration.

Gd-DTPA has been studied in several experimental models of myocardial ischemia that primarily differ from each other in the duration of coronary artery ligation, the time period between contrast administration and imaging, and the presence or absence of reperfusion [55–59]. These experimental studies using Gd-DTPA demonstrated that changes in relaxation times already occur very early (2 minutes) after coronary artery occlusion, implying that Gd-DTPA allows the detection of early myocardial ischemia even before the onset of myocardial edema formation or the development of irreversible damage. These studies also suggest that Gd-DTPA may be useful to outline distribution of regional myocardial blood flow.

In a study by Miller *et al.* [60], using MR imaging, it was possible to measure myocardial flow reserve during pharmacologic dilatation by dipyridamole. There was a significant correlation between changes in Gd-DTPA enhanced MR signal and microsphere myocardial blood flow. Further experimental studies have shown that the use of Gd-DTPA may discriminate between occlusive and reperfused infarcts based on differences in signal intensities [61–64]. Moreover, administration of Gd-DTPA early after reperfusion allowed the identification of the area at risk by selective concentration of Gd-DTPA in reperfused myocardium [65]. Holman *et al.* [66], in 21 isolated rat hearts, compared distribution of Evans blue staining and Gd-DTPA enhancement in ischemic and reperfused myocardium, and showed the excellent capability of Gd-DTPA to identify ischemia and reperfusion by contrast enhancement (Figure 7.3). Nishimura *et al.* [67] measured infarct size both by MR imaging using Gd-DTPA and indium-111 labeled antimyosin. Gd-DTPA showed significant contrast enhancement of the infarcted area and the extent of the contrast enhancement expressed infarct size precisely. Van Dijkman *et al.* [68] showed that gadolinium-enhanced MR imaging identified infarcted myocardium with great sensitivity in an *in vivo* porcine model.

In summary, Gd-DTPA enhanced MR imaging experimentally demonstrated that changes in relaxation times occur very early (2 minutes) after coronary artery occlusion, implying that Gd-DTPA allows the detection of early myocardial ischemia even before the onset of myocardial edema formation or the development of irreversible damage. These studies also suggest that Gd-DTPA may be useful to outline the distribution of regional myocardial perfusion under various (patho)physiological conditions, and to distinguish between viable and nonviable myocardium.

Clinical studies with Gd-DTPA

In recent years, several clinical studies with Gd-DTPA have been performed. Eichstaedt *et al.* [69] were the first to show, in 26 patients with acute myocardial infarction, that 11 patients, who were studied with Gd-DTPA 5 to 10 days after the acute event, had a 70% average increase of signal intensity within zones of infarcted myocardium, while only a 20% increase of signal intensity in normal myocardial tissue was observed. The other 15 patients were imaged later in the course of infarction and did not show differences in intensity ratio between infarcted and normal tissue. These findings were corroborated in a recent report by Nishimura *et al.* [70] who studied 17 infarct patients with MR imaging and Gd-DTPA at an average of 5, 12, 30, and 90 days after the acute event. Increased signal intensity in the infarcted area was observed at 5 and 12 days, implying that only acute (or subacute) myocardial infarcts show significant accumulation of Gd-DTPA. De Roos *et al.* [71] showed, in five patients using MR imaging with Gd-DTPA 2 to 17 days after myocardial infarction, that the signal intensity of infarcted versus normal myocardium was significantly greater after Gd-DTPA administration than before Gd-DTPA, both by visual and computer-assessed analysis. The use of Gd-DTPA-improved infarct definition obviated the need for multi-echo imaging techniques. This study was extended to 20 patients with acute myocardial infarction and showed maximal contrast 20–25 minutes after administration of Gd-DTPA (Figure 7.4) [72–74]. Moreover, a significant correlation between electrocardiographic infarct site and local increase of signal intensity based on region of interest analysis was observed. In 25 patients, 10 of whom were studied within 72 hours after myocardial infarction, van Dijkman *et al.* [73] showed that signal intensity of Gd-DTPA was significantly increased in the infarcted areas of the 15 patients who were studied more than 72 hours after the acute onset, indicating increased accumulation of Gd-DTPA in a more advanced stage of the disease process. In a larger study by Van Dijkman *et al.* [75], in 84 patients with acute myocardial infarction, it was shown that Gd-DTPA enhancement improved visualization of infarcted areas up to 6 weeks after onset of symptoms and had a maximal effect within 1 week after infarction. Holman *et al.* [76] showed a high correlation (r=0.93) between infarct size measured with gadolinium-enhanced MR imaging and enzymatically determined infarct size in patients 3 to 7 days after the acute event (Figure 7.5).

These encouraging results have led to the initiation of clinical studies to determine whether the use of Gd-DTPA allows the discrimination of reperfused versus non-reperfused myocardial areas. In an initial report by van der Wall *et al.* [77], it was shown that signal intensities do not differ between reperfused and non-reperfused myocardial areas. However, in a study by de Roos *et al.* [78] it was observed that the morphological appearance of contrast enhancement by Gd-DTPA may provide some clues as to the presence or absence of reperfusion; reperfusion goes along with a homogeneous aspect, while lack of reperfusion may be visualized as a heterogeneous enhancement of contrast.

Apart from these morphologic characteristics, de Roos *et al.* [79] used MR imaging with Gd-DTPA to show that infarct size was significantly smaller in patients with documented reperfusion than in patients without reperfusion (Figure 7.6).

In summary, the use of paramagnetic contrast agents has considerably improved the detection of myocardial infarction. Particularly in patients within 1 week following myocardial infarction, infarct size can be accurately measured using Gd-DTPA-enhanced MR imaging and the effect of interventional therapy can be assessed.

Ultrafast MR imaging

Recently, ultrafast gradient-echo sequences, called subsecond MR imaging or high-speed MR imaging, have become available which require a fraction of a

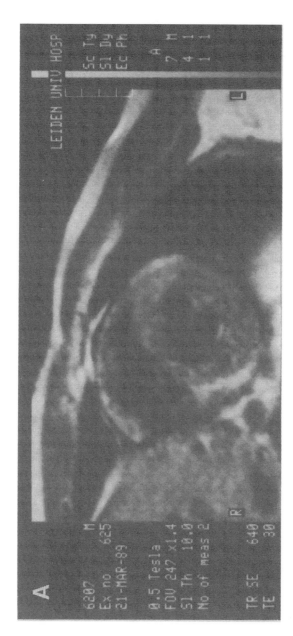

Figure 7.4.A. Cardiac MR image of patient with anteroseptal wall infarction before administration of Gd-DTPA.

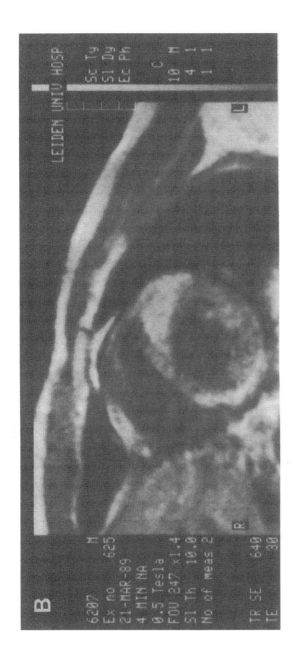

Figure 7.4B. Cardiac MR image of patient with anteroseptal wall infarction 20 to 25 minutes after administration of Gd-DTPA. Contrast enhancement is visible in anteroseptal areas with extension to apex.

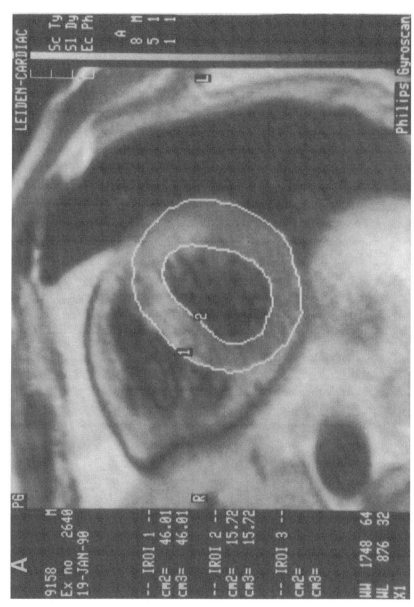

Figure 7.5A. Computer-constructed contours of subepicardial (1) and subendocardial (2) borders on MR image after administration of Gd-DTPA in patient with anterior wall infarction.

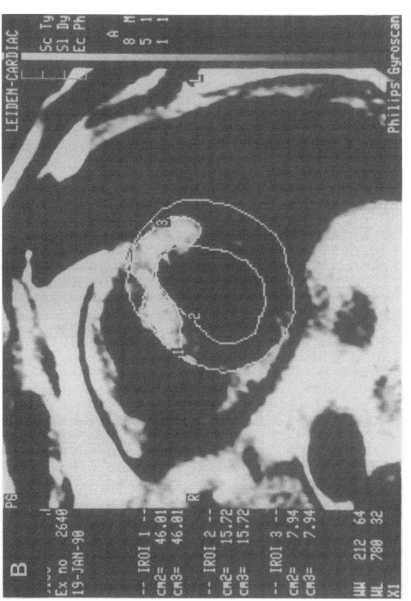

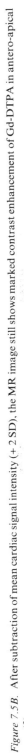

Figure 7.5B. After subtraction of mean cardiac signal intensity (+ 2 SD), the MR image still shows marked contrast enhancement of Gd-DTPA in antero-apical area (3).

C

Anterior view

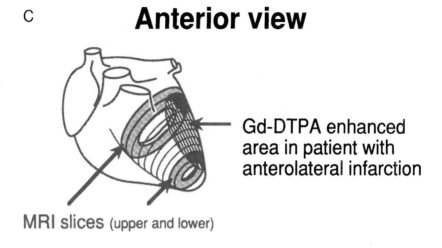

Gd-DTPA enhanced
area in patient with
anterolateral infarction

MRI slices (upper and lower)

Figure 7.5C. Summing up the extent of contrast enhancement in the different tomographic slices covering the complete left ventricle, an estimate of infarct size can be obtained.

D

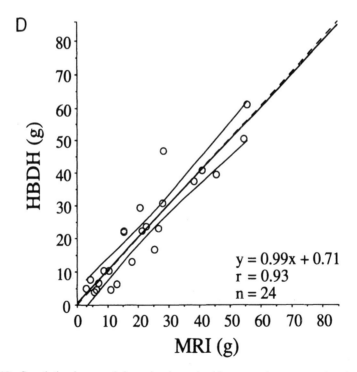

Figure 7.5D. Correlation between infarct size determined by magnetic resonance imaging (MRI) and enzymatic infarct size calculated from cumulative release of alpha-hydroxybutyrate dehydrogenase (HBDH) activity in plasma. Indicated are regression line and 95% confidence interval. Note that line of identity (dashed line) is within 95% confidence interval. (Reproduced with permission, from Holman *et al.* [76].)

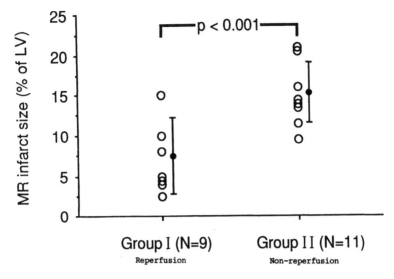

Figure 7.6. Following successful reperfusion a significant reduction of magnetic resonance imaging (MR)-determined infarct size is observed. Infarct size was calculated from the percentage of left ventricular myocardium that showed contrast enhancement following Gd-DTPA administration. (Reproduced with permission, from de Roos *et al.* [79].)

second for data acquisition [80–82]. Coupled with the bolus administration of contrast media and the acquisition of first-pass images of the left ventricular myocardium, ultrafast MR imaging has great potential in the assessment of regional myocardial perfusion (Figure 7.7). The technique has advantages over conventional methods such as higher spatial resolution and a reduction of attenuation problems related to patient motion during the imaging procedure, as a result of the short duration of the procedure. This improves patient comfort and facilitates the study of large patient groups. In addition, ultrafast imaging enables the study of fast physiological processes, such as cardiac first-pass effects. Two current limitations of the technique are its reliance on a T1 effect and its ability to acquire images at only one or two levels during a single bolus injection. Although future software improvements may allow for more tomographic sections to be acquired at several levels with each heart beat, echo-planar imaging may more easily allow multiple myocardial levels to be imaged during the first pass of a contrast agent.

Experimental and clinical studies with ultrafast MR imaging

Atkinson *et al.* [83] demonstrated that a T1-weighted ultrafast imaging technique can provide adequate temporal and spatial resolution to permit first-pass perfusion studies of the heart. In an occlusive infarct model that used an isolated perfused rat heart, marked differences in contrast enhancement were observed between perfused and nonperfused segments. In studies of human subjects, it was possible to dynamically show the first-pass transit of a Gd-DTPA bolus, administered in a peripheral vein, through the four cardiac

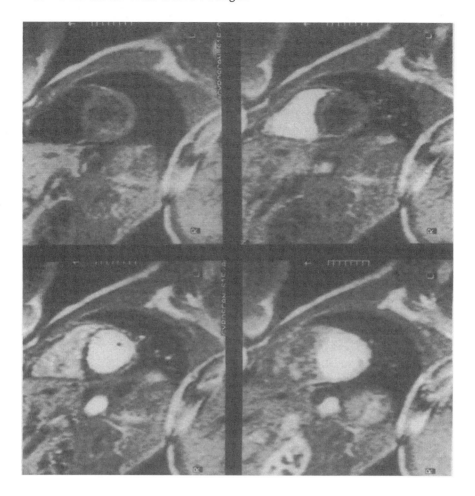

Figure 7.7. Baseline MR image (upper left panel) and MR images of sequential signal enhancement following administration of Gd-DTPA in the right ventricular (RV) cavity (upper right panel), the pulmonary vasculature, the left ventricular (LV) cavity and the aorta (lower left panel), and the myocardium (lower right panel). (Reproduced with permission, from Van Rugge *et al.* [85].)

chambers and into the left ventricular myocardium. In the perfused rat heart model and in humans, these wash-in effects of Gd-DTPA occurred during several seconds.

Manning *et al.* [84] used ultrafast MRI for the assessment of coronary stenosis in patients with chest pain. Regional myocardium perfused by a diseased vessel demonstrated a lower peak signal intensity and lower rate of signal increase than did myocardium perfused by coronary arteries without stenosis. Repeat MRI study after revascularization showed an increase in peak signal intensity. The patients with an area of myocardium perfused by a diseased vessel and associated low peak signal intensity had the greatest improvement in regional peak signal intensity after revascularization.

Van Rugge *et al.* evaluated the ultrafast MRI for the assessment of dynamic contrast enhancement and myocardial perfusion abnormalities in 7 healthy volunteers [85] and 20 patients after myocardial infarction [86]. After Gd-DTPA administration, infarcted myocardium demonstrated a signal intensity enhancement of 50%, whereas in normal myocardium an enhancement of 134% was obtained. Ultrafast MRI using gadolinium-DTPA clearly identified myocardial perfusion abnormalities in patients after myocardial infarction (Figure 7.8). The infarct site on MRI corresponded with the location of wall motion asynergy determined by echocardiography. It was concluded that gadolinium-DTPA-enhanced ultrafast MRI provides non-invasive assessment of myocardial perfusion in patients with proven coronary artery disease.

To summarize, ultrafast MRI provides the opportunity to acquire dynamic information related to passage of a contrast agent through the coronary circulation and, thus, provides an indirect measure of myocardial perfusion. Applying this technique to patients at rest, myocardial regions perfused by a severely stenosed coronary artery can be detected by a delayed increase in signal intensity and a decreased peak signal intensity. In this way, performed both at rest and in combination with dipyridamole, ultrafast MR imaging may become a good clinical marker of myocardial viability.

Cardiac wall motion

Cine MR imaging

By assessing wall motion dynamics, cine MR imaging can be considered as the next standard of viability. The temporal resolution attained by cine MR imaging has extended the application of MR imaging to the assessment of cardiac function [87–89]. Cine MR imaging can be performed sequentially, so that the severity of cardiac disease states can be monitored and the response to interventions determined. Since both the endocardial and epicardial borders are well defined by MR imaging, it is possible to assess wall thickening during the cardiac cycle and detect regional myocardial dysfunction (Figure 7.9) [90,91]. The cinematic display of MR images facilitates identification of abnormal wall motion during the cardiac cycle. Regions with previous myocardial infarcts exhibit absent or severely reduced wall thickening during systole [92]. Although there may be normal systolic inward motion, the absence of wall thickening indicates that the infarcted region is only passively pulled inward by traction of the surrounding normal myocardium [93].

The capability of MR imaging to provide sequential information about the state of pathologically altered myocardium in combination with assessment of diastolic wall thickness and systolic wall thickening, makes it suitable for identification of viable myocardium in areas previously affected by myocardial infarction. Data from Baer *et al.* [94], who compared wall thickness measurements by cine MR imaging with technetium-99m MIBI tomographic

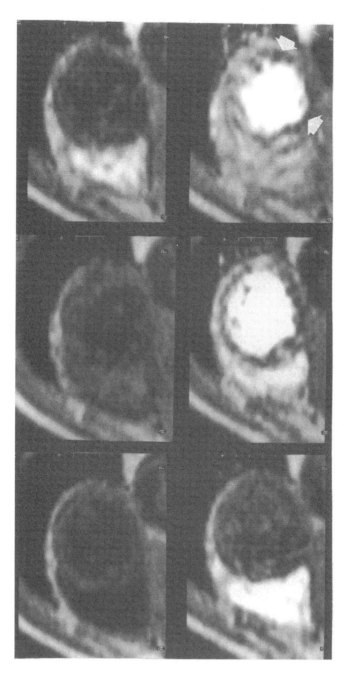

Figure 7.8: Series of 6 sequential ultrafast short-axis MR images following bolus administration of Gd-DTPA in a patient with healed myocardial infarction of the inferior wall. Ultimately, a decreased signal density is observed in the infarcted inferior myocardial area (arrows), compared to the normal anterior wall. (Reproduced with permission, from Van Rugge *et al.* [86].)

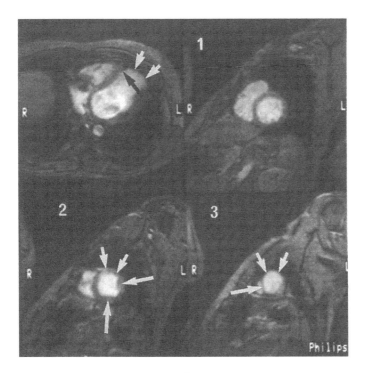

Figure 7.9. Diastolic gradient-echo MR images of a patient with a large transmural myocardial infarction. Upper left) Severe thinning of the anterior wall (small white arrows) and the anterior portion of the interventricular septum (small black arrow) is evident on this transverse section through the left ventricle, slightly below the inferior portion of the mitral valve ring. Upper right) The most posterior short-axis section (1), close to the mitral valve plane, demonstrates homogeneous and normal wall thickness throughout the entire circumference of the left ventricle. Lower left) The midventricular short axis section (2), at the level of papillary muscles (large white arrows), shows some thinning of the anterior wall (small white arrows) with preserved septal thickness. Lower right) Anterior wall (small white arrows) and interventricular septum (long white arrow) are maximally thinned on this apical short axis section (3). (Reproduced with permission, from Sechtem *et al.* [9].)

imaging, showed a high concordance in patients with large chronic Q-wave infarcts (Figure 7.10). However, Perrone-Filardi *et al.* [95,96], using positron emission tomography, showed the presence of metabolic activity in many regions with reduced end diastolic wall thickness and absent wall thickening. This indicates that the assessment of regional anatomy and function may be suboptimal in distinguishing asynergic but viable myocardium from nonviable myocardium. Further studies are needed to clarify these differences.

Dobutamine stress cine MR imaging

Early manifestations of coronary artery disease can be studied with dobutamine stress cine MR imaging [97]. Development of stress-induced wall motion

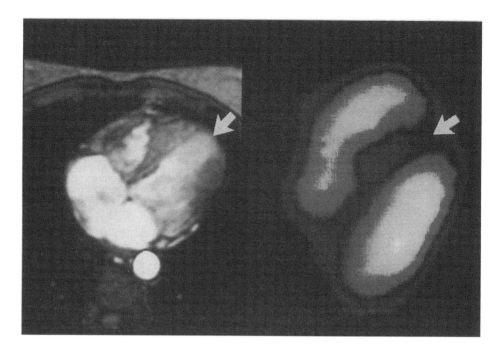

Figure 7.10. Corresponding gradient-echo MR image (left) and MIBI-SPECT image (right) obtained from the patient described in Figure 7.9. The zone of severe wall thinning seen on the MR image (arrow) corresponds exactly to the region with severely reduced technetium-99m MIBI-uptake (arrow). (Reproduced with permission, from Sechtem *et al.* [9].)

abnormalities is an early and reliable sign of myocardial ischemia, preceding electrocardiographic changes and angina. As physical exercise during MR imaging is difficult due to motion artifacts and space restriction, it is more practical to induce stress using pharmacologic stress agents. In this respect, dobutamine appears the most appropriate agent for eliciting wall motion abnormalities [98].

Van Rugge *et al.* [99] clearly identified wall motion dynamics in 23 healthyvolunteers, and provided calculations of segmental wall thickening and hemodynamic parameters using dobutamine stress imaging. In 37 patients with

Figure 7.11. A) Short-axis MR scan during peak dobutamine stress end-systole in a patient with ▶ two-vessel coronary artery disease (left anterior descending and right coronary artery). Endocardial and epicardial contours are depicted in green, the centerline in red, and the chords in blue. Chord 1 is located at the inner posterior junction between the right ventricular wall and the interventricular septum followed by clockwise numbering. Note the decreased systolic wall thickening at the posterior wall.

B) The shaded area represents normal mean percent wall thickening (% wth) ± 2SD during peak dobutamine stress: the continuous black line represents the percent systolic wall thickening of the patient. Note the decreased wall thickening between chords 86 and 100, corresponding with the posterior wall. Also between chords 23 and 26, corresponding with the anteroseptal wall, minimally decreased wall thickening is observed. (Courtesy of Van Rugge) coronary artery disease, Van Rugge *et al.* [100] showed an overall sensitivity of 81% and a specificity of 100% when using dobutamine MR imaging; in patients with single-, double-, and triple-vessel disease, the sensitivity values were 75%, 80% and 100%, respectively. In a subsequent study, in 39 consecutive patients

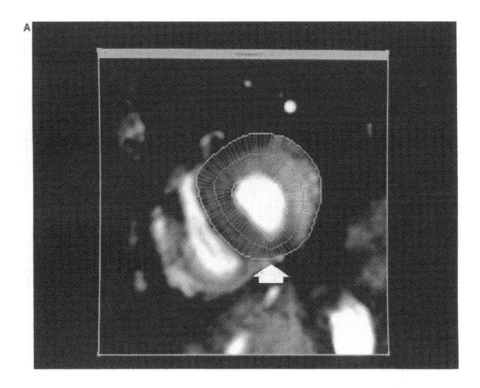

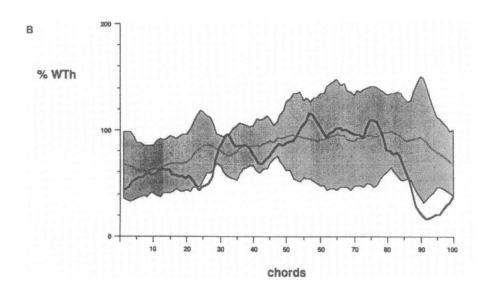

with clinically suspected coronary artery disease referred for coronary arteriography, and in 10 normal volunteers, it was shown that dobutamine MRI clearly identified wall motion abnormalities by quantitative analysis using the centerline method (Figure 7.11); the sensitivity, specificity, and accuracy were 91%, 80%, and 90%, respectively [101].

To summarize, cine MR – particularly using dobutamine stress – may constitute an adequate technique for detecting myocardial viability. Regions with previous myocardial infarction show reduced enddiastolic wall thickness and absent or severely reduced wall thickening during systole. In theory, these aspects make cine MR imaging a well-suited technique for differentiating viable myocardium from nonviable myocardium in areas previously affected by myocardial infarction. However, the presence of metabolic activity in some regions with abnormal wall motion implies that this method might not be very accurate. Therefore, optimal viability assessment in infarcted areas by cine MR imaging should be used in conjunction with other imaging modalities, such as thallium-201 scintigraphy and positron emission tomography, to allow for a precise distinction between viable and nonviable myocardium.

Myocardial tagging

Myocardial tagging, a recently developed technique, permits determination of the absolute motion and thickening of specific myocardial segments [102,103]. This can be used to evaluate myocardial rotational deformation [104,105] and differences in subendocardial and epicardial wall motion [106]. It is likely that this method will become the reference standard for assessments of wall motion and wall thickening and, hence, viability in the setting of acute myocardial infarction.

Cardiac metabolism

MR spectroscopy

MR spectroscopy can be considered as the third MR standard of myocardial viability. Using phosphorus-31 (31-P) MR spectroscopy, changes in the high-energy phosphate metabolism of myocardial cells resulting from ischemia or infarction can be studied [107,108]. With MR spectroscopy one can determine the concentration and kinetics of metabolically important compounds, measure intracellular pH, and establish the fate of exogenously administered tracers. Three-dimensionally localized 31-P spectra are obtained from the myocardium using a surface coil placed on the chest over the cardiac apex (Figure 7.12). The spectrum provides quantifiable information regarding the concentration of multiple metabolic high-energy phosphate compounds [109]. Cardiac 31-P spectra disclose metabolites such as inorganic phosphate (Pi), phospho-monoesters, phosphodiesters, phosphocreatine (PCr), and 3 peaks from

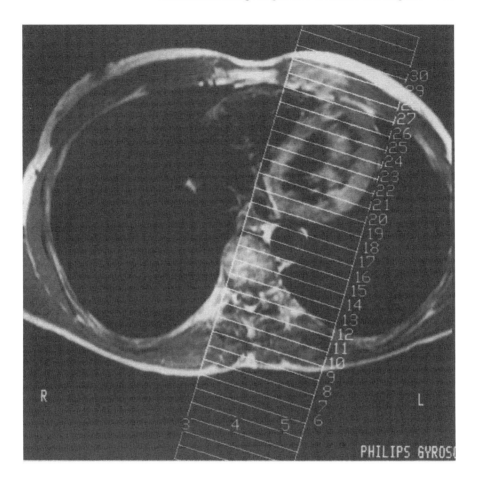

Figure 7.12. Transverse spin-echo image through the chest wall and left ventricle demonstrates a series of 1-cm-thick sections from which P-31 MR spectra were collected with a 10-cm-diameter surface coil. Note angulation of the section column with respect to the left ventricular wall to optimize the spatial relationship. (Reproduced with permission, from de Roos *et al.* [109].)

adenosine triphosphate (ATP) (Figure 7.13). The phosphomonoester region often includes 2,3-diphosphoglycerate, which is present in the blood pool of cardiac chambers and myocardium, overlapping the inorganic phosphate peak. Furthermore, it is technically difficult to separate myocardial signals from those of the chest wall muscle and the nearby blood pool. However, when the inorganic phosphate peak is resolved, the intracellular pH of the myocardium can be estimated from the distance between the peaks of Pi and PCr. The ratio between phosphocreatine and inorganic phosphate is an indicator of the energy reserve of the heart, and this ratio will promptly change when ischemia develops.

With the reduction of myocardial blood flow, myocardial contraction of the

³¹P MR Heart Spectrum: Normal Volunteer
One Dimensional Phase Encoding and Column Selection

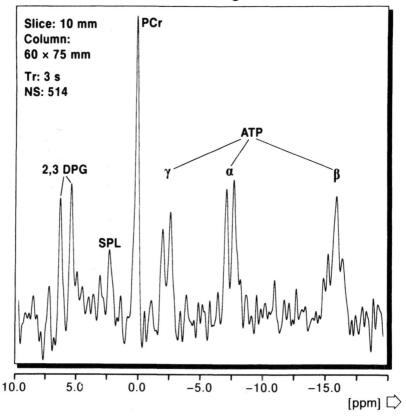

Slice: 10 mm
Column:
60 × 75 mm

Tr: 3 s
NS: 514

PCr

ATP

2,3 DPG

γ   α   β

SPL

10.0   5.0   0.0   −5.0   −10.0   −15.0

[ppm] ⇨

Figure 7.13. Phosphorus-31 spectrum from the human heart obtained with proton-decoupled 31P MR spectroscopy using image selected *in vivo* spectroscopy (ISIS) at 1.5 T (Philips Gyroscan S15, Best, The Netherlands). Note resonance from 2,3-diphosphoglycerate (DPG) contained in blood, serum phospholipids (SPL) phosphocreatine (PCr), and the three peaks from adenosine triphosphate (ATP). (Reproduced with permission, from de Roos *et al.* [108].)

affected segment will cease, accompanied by a rapid fall in phosphocreatine, a rise in inorganic phosphate and a fall in tissue pH, while the ATP levels are maintained until phosphocreatine is depleted. 31-P MR spectroscopy can detect myocardial ischemia and infarction by profound changes in high-energy phosphate compounds. Theoretically, necrotic myocardium should not contain any PCr or ATP. This allows differentiation from partially infarcted myocardium with viable cells that do contain PCr or ATP. Studies performed using P-31 MR spectroscopy suggest that it may be possible to differentiate reversibly from irreversibly injured myocardium [110]. Although the results of these studies are encouraging, a number of technical problems must be addressed to allow these studies to become clinically applicable. The technical problems relate primarily to the relatively low concentrations of the nuclei being observed, which makes the signal weak. This limits spatial resolution and prolongs study time.

It is important to recognize that the nature of the information derived from 31-P MR spectroscopy is fundamentally different from that obtained from proton imaging. In MR spectroscopy, stronger and more uniform magnetic fields are applied than in MR imaging, so that the signals from individual chemicals are resolved.

Most of the research on cardiac MR spectroscopy has been directed towards detection of myocardial ischemia. Spectroscopic investigation of ischemia and infarction have ranged from analyses of myocardial tissue samples to image-guided *in vivo* studies of intact animals and humans. The latter studies have non-invasively shown metabolic alteration due to myocardial ischemia, thus confirming the feasibility of clinical cardiac MR spectroscopy.

Thrombolytic therapy, coronary angioplasty, and other means of re-establishing blood flow to ischemic myocardium have become increasingly prevalent in recent years. The success of these techniques underscores the clinical need for a reliable method of assessing myocardial viability, the effects of reperfusion, and the recovery of myocardial physiologic function after re-establishment of coronary blood flow. Although MR spectroscopy may be useful in this regard, the task is complicated by the fact that ischemic regions of myocardium are histologically heterogeneous, containing cells with different degrees of ischemic damage. MR spectroscopy may be useful to quantify and characterize ischemic myocardium in relatively stable patients with coronary artery disease, particularly those in whom the severity of disease is out of proportion to clinical symptoms.

Experimental studies

From studies on isolated and surgically exposed animal hearts, it has been shown that the onset of severe ischemia is associated with an early change in high-energy phosphate metabolism with a decrease in PCr and in the ratio PCr/ATP [111–113].

After reperfusion, viable myocardium can be detected from an overshoot in PCr concentration [114–117]. The origin of that overshoot is likely multifactorial, and reduction in energy requirements resulting from the reduced contractility (stunning) of the reperfused myocardium is believed to be important [116,117]. The pH normalizes upon reperfusion, whether or not the reperfused myocardium is viable, and therefore pH is not a reliable measure of viability. Similarly, the Pi concentration decreases upon reperfusion, whether or not tissue viability is preserved, and is also not a useful indicator. It is likely that the effects of reperfusion on pH an Pi levels represent, in part, washout of protons and Pi, respectively, from the risk zone upon reperfusion.

Rehr *et al.* [110] confirmed these data, using MR spectroscopy to make a distinction between reperfused-viable and reperfused-infarcted myocardium in a canine model of acute coronary occlusion. *In vivo* myocardial pH and PCr, ATP, and Pi levels were measured at baseline and for the first 90 minutes after reperfusion of a total coronary artery occlusion producing either predominantly viable (9 animals) or infarcted (9 animals) myocardium in the region of metabolic study. Myocardial viability was assessed in each animal by means of postmortem triphenyltetrazolium chloride staining. Tissue was characterized from the *in vivo* P-31 MR data by means of logistic regression analysis. The accuracy of using the P-31 MR data for distinguishing reperfused-viable from reperfused-infarcted myocardium was 100%. Results of the logistic regression procedure indicated that PCr was the metabolic variable enabling the most effective separation of reperfused-viable and reperfused-infarcted myocardium. Thus, metabolic data obtained with P-31 MR spectroscopy permit effective separation of reperfused-viable from reperfused-infarcted myocardium [110].

Wroblewski *et al.* [118] showed that the existence of graded metabolic recovery in rabbits was dependent upon the severity of the ischemic insult, and the correlations observed suggested that metabolic data may indicate tissue viability. Significant correlations were found between PCr and Pi reperfusion values and myocardial viability (Figure 7.14).

Rehr *et al.* [119] studied the ability of *in vivo* P-31 nuclear magnetic resonance spectroscopy to distinguish reperfused-viable (stunned) from reperfused-

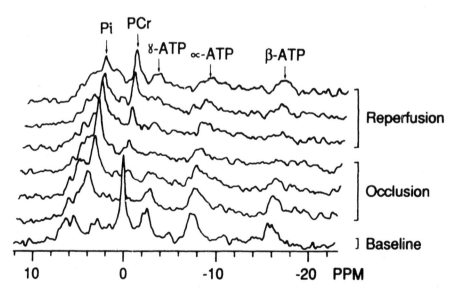

Figure 7.14. Stacked plot of MR spectroscopy data over time for eight rabbit hearts, who underwent 30 minutes of coronary occlusion followed by reperfusion. The figure shows seven spectra; one baseline, three ischemic, and three reperfusion spectra, which correspond to 10, 20, and 30 minutes of occlusion, and 10, 20, and 30 minutes of reperfusion. During occlusion a fall in phosphocreatine (PCr) and adenosine triphosphate (ATP) levels is noticed together with a rise in inorganic phosphate (Pi), which is restored rapidly following reperfusion. (Reproduced with permission, from Wroblewski *et al.* [118].)

infarcted myocardium at 6, 30, and 54 hours, following coronary artery occlusion in a canine model. A 15-minute occlusion produced reperfused-viable myocardium in 5 animals and a 360-minute occlusion produced reperfused-infarcted myocardium in 6 animals. The post-reperfusion risk zone showed a significantly reduced PCr concentration throughout the 3-day study period in infarcted but nonviable myocardium. The post-reperfusion ratio, Pi/PCr, as determined by MR spectroscopy, was elevated throughout the study period in infarcted but not in viable reperfused myocardium. Post-reperfusion Pi concentration was elevated at 6 hours, but not subsequently in reperfused-infarcted myocardium, and was not elevated in reperfused-viable myocardium. Logistic regression models selected PCr concentration and the Pi/PCr ratio as providing the best discrimination between reperfused-viable and reperfused-infarcted myocardium. After reperfusion, viable tissue is associated with a high PCr and a low Pi/PCr ratio in contrast to nonviable (infarcted) tissue that is associated with a low PCr and a high Pi/PCr ratio. The accuracy of P-31 MR variables selected by logistic regression analysis for determining myocardial viability ranged from 97% to 100%.

In conclusion, these experimental studies indicated that 1) myocardial ischemia is associated with a decreased PCr/ATP ratio and 2) a high PCr concentration and a low Pi/PCr ratio are reliable indicators of viability, in distinguishing viable from nonviable myocardium after reperfusion.

Clinical studies

The few human studies performed with MR spectroscopy have been focused on the changes during ischemia and have used the PCr/ATP ratio as a measure of metabolic response to ischemia. Difficulties of spatial localization have limited the number of cardiac studies using 31-P MR in humans. However, several investigators have shown the feasibility and potential of this technique in selected circumstances.

The diagnosis of myocardial ischemia with phosphorus-31 MR in humans has been limited by the inability to accurately measure myocardial Pi, due to the overlapping signal from the 2,3-diphosphoglycerate of chamber blood. Thus, calculation of the ratio PCr/Pi, shown previously to be a sensitive marker of ischemia, is difficult in humans [120–127]. Therefore, in most studies, the PCr/ATP ratio is used as a marker for ischemia and infarction. However, due to differences in applied techniques, like DRESS (depth-resolved surface coil spectroscopy) and ISIS (image-selected *in vivo* spectroscopy), the PCr/ATP ratio exhibits a wide range of normal values, from 0.89 to 1.93, which makes distinction from diseased myocardium difficult.

In normal individuals, Bottomley *et al.* [128] first demonstrated the capability of measuring cardiac PCr and ATP. The authors calculated a PCr/ATP ratio of 1.3, which was in agreement with earlier values in animal hearts. In human hearts, 5 to 9 days post-myocardial infarction, a low PCr/ATP ratio (approximately 1.1), and elevated Pi levels in some spectra were observed, in regions that might correspond with the infarcted region [129]. Blackledge *et al.* [121] found a PCr/ATP ratio of 1.55 in 6 normal subjects. Schaefer *et al.* [127] used image-selected *in vivo* spectroscopy, a technique that allows three-dimensional localization of the volume of interest. They found, in 12 young healthy volunteers, a PCr/ATP ratio of 1.33.

Weiss *et al.* [122] studied regional myocardial metabolism of high-energy phosphates during isometric exercise in patients with coronary artery disease. At rest, the PCr/ATP ratio in the left ventricle was 1.72 in 11 normal subjects as compared to 1.45 in 16 patients with coronary artery disease. During exercise, this ratio did not change in the normal group, but changed considerably to 0.91 in the group with coronary artery disease and recovered to 1.27 two minutes after exercise. Only 3 patients with coronary artery disease had clinical symptoms during exercise. Repeat exercise testing in 5 patients after revascularization yielded values of 1.60 at rest and 1.62 during exercise, as compared to 1.51 at rest and 1.02 during exercise before revascularization. It can be concluded that the decrease in PCr/ATP ratio reflects a transient imbalance between oxygen supply and demand in myocardium with compromised blood flow. Exercise testing with 31-P MR spectroscopy seems to be a useful method of assessing the effect of ischemia on myocardial metabolism of high-energy phosphates and of monitoring the response to treatment.

To summarize, MR spectroscopy has established itself clearly as an important investigative tool for the study of cardiac metabolism and energetics. In animal models, it can provide insight into basic metabolic processes in both health and disease. Its non-invasive nature and capacity for serial measurements in the same system allow changes in biologic systems to be monitored over time, while its ability to measure different nuclei and, hence, different metabolic processes gives MR spectroscopy immense flexibility.

In relative contrast to animal studies, human cardiac MR spectroscopy is in its infancy. To date, cardiac 31-P spectroscopy has been successfully implemented in only a few centers. These studies have primarily examined normal subjects to establish the feasibility of such examinations with a variety of techniques. The few reports of metabolic abnormalities detected by 31-P MRS have been limited by problems of accurate spatial localization and large sample volumes. The ultimate utility of human spectroscopy with phosphorus or any other nucleus will depend on the success of efforts to increase the sensitivity and spatial selectivity of the MR spectroscopy experiment. These efforts include utilizing systems of higher field strength and homogeneity, as well as improving pulse sequences and radiofrequency coil designs. In addition, the demonstration of some degree of sensitivity and specificity of metabolic abnormalities in disease states will be necessary before clinical use is indicated. If these requirements are met, human cardiac spectroscopy may provide useful information about cardiac metabolic processes (and thus viability) and, combined with proton MR imaging, may enable complete non-invasive evaluation with one technology. The rapid advances over the past few years attest to the feasibility of this goal.

Conclusion

The unique features of MR techniques, such as good anatomical and temporal resolution, three-dimensional capabilities, easy reproducibility, an unlimited field of view and lack of radiation, and the possibility of *in vivo* measurement of myocardial biochemistry, render the MR techniques a modality especially suited for determination of myocardial viability in patients with coronary artery disease. To date, MR techniques are only sparsely used for this purpose. This results from long scanning times and relatively high costs of the equipment. Recent developments, like high speed subsecond imaging will have a significant impact on the time required for the study and will potentially reduce costs. So far, MR imaging techniques may prove valuable in the detection of a wide range of pathophysiological entities, such as flow and perfusion, wall motion, and cardiac metabolism. This will give the MR techniques a growing role in the determination of viability in patients with coronary artery disease.

References

1. van der Wall EE, De Roos A (eds). Magnetic Resonance Imaging in Coronary Artery Disease. Dordrecht: Kluwer Academic Publishers 1991.
2. van der Wall EE, De Roos A, Van Voorthuisen AE, Bruschke AVG. Magnetic resonance imaging: A new approach for evaluating coronary artery disease? Am Heart J 1991; 121: 1203–20.
3. Rahimtoola SH. A perspective on the three large multicenter randomized clinical trials of coronary bypass surgery for chronic stable angina. Circulation 1985; 72: V123–35.
4. Bodenheimer MM, Banka VS, Hermann GA, Trout RG, Pasdar H, Helfant RH. Reversible asynergy. Histopathologic and electrocardiographic correlations in patients with coronary artery disease. Circulation 1976; 53: 792–6.
5. Chatterjee K, Swann HJ, Parmley WW, Sustaita H, Marcus HS, Matloff J. Influence of direct myocardial revascularization on left ventricular asynergy and function in patients with coronary heart disease and with and without previous myocardial infarction. Circulation 1973; 47: 276–86.
6. Braunwald E, Kloner RA. The stunned myocardium: Prolonged, postischemic ventricular dysfunction. Circulation 1982; 66: 1146–49.
7. Iskandrian AS, Heo J, Helfant RH, Segal BL. Chronic myocardial ischemia and left ventricular function. Ann Intern Med 1987; 107: 925–7.
8. Peshock RM. Assessing myocardial viability with magnetic resonance imaging. Am J Card Imaging 1992; 6: 237–43.
9. Sechtem U, Voth E, Baer F, Schneider C, Theissen P, Schicha H. Assessment of residual viability in patients with myocardial infarction using magnetic resonance techniques. Int J Card Imaging 1993; 9 (Suppl 1): 31–40.
10. Williams ES, Kaplan JI, Thatcher F, Zimmerman G, Knoebel SB. Prolongation of proton spin lattice relaxation times in regionally ischemic tissue from dog hearts. J Nucl Med 1980; 21: 449–53.
11. Higgins CB, Herfkins R, Lipton MJ, Sievers R, Sheldon P, Kaufman L *et al.* Nuclear magnetic resonance imaging of acute myocardial infarction in dogs: Alterations in magnetic relaxation times. Am J Cardiol 1983; 52: 184–8.
12. Pflugfelder PW, Wisenberg G, Prato FS, Carroll SE. Serial imaging of canine myocardial infarction by *in vivo* nuclear magnetic resonance. J Am Coll Cardiol 1986; 7: 843–9.

13. Ratner AV, Okada RD, Newell JB, Pohost GM. The relationship between proton nuclear magnetic resonance relaxation parameters and myocardial perfusion with acute coronary arterial occlusion and reperfusion. Circulation 1985; 71: 823–8.

14. Johnston DL, Brady TJ, Ratner AV, Rosen BR, Newell JB, Pohost GM *et al.* Assessment of myocardial ischemia with proton magnetic resonance: Effects of a three hour coronary occlusion with and without reperfusion. Circulation 1985; 71: 595–601.

15. Slutsky RA, Brown JJ, Peck WW, Stritch G, Andre MP. Effects of transient coronary ischemia and reperfusion on myocardial edema formation and *in vitro* magnetic relaxation times [retracted in: J Am Coll Cardiol 1987; 9: 973]. J Am Coll Cardiol 1984; 3: 1454–60.

16. Aisen AM, Buda AJ, Zotz RJ, Buckwalter KA. Visualization of myocardial infarction and subsequent coronary reperfusion with MRI using a dog model. Magn Reson Imaging 1987; 5: 399–404.

17. Johnston DL, Liu P, Rosen BR, Levine RA, Beaulieu PA, Brady TJ *et al. In vivo* detection of reperfused myocardium by nuclear magnetic resonance imaging. J Am Coll Cardiol 1987; 9: 127–35.

18. Miller DD, Johnston DL, Dragotakes D, Newell JB, Aretz T, Kantor HL *et al.* Effect of hyperosmotic mannitol on magnetic resonance relaxation parameters in reperfused canine myocardial infarction. Magn Reson Imaging 1989; 7: 79–88.

19. Tscholakoff D, Higgins CB, Sechtem U, Caputo G, Derugin N. MRI of reperfused myocardial infarct in dogs. AJR Am J Roentgenol 1986; 146: 925–30.

20. Buda AJ, Aisen AM, Juni JE, Gallagher KP, Zotz RJ. Detection and sizing of myocardial ischemia and infarction by nuclear magnetic resonance imaging in the canine heart. Am Heart J 1985; 110: 1284–90.

21. Rokey R, Verani MS, Bolli R, Kuo LC, Ford JJ, Wendt RE *et al.* Myocardial infarct size quantification by MR imaging early after coronary artery occlusion in dogs. Radiology 1986; 158: 771–4.

22. Bouchard A, Reeves RC, Cranney G, Bishop SP, Pohost GM, Assessment of myocardial infarct size by means of T_2-weighted ^1H nuclear magnetic resonance imaging. Am Heart J 1989; 117: 281–9.

23. Wisenberg G, Prato FS, Carroll SE, Turner KL, Marshall T. Serial nuclear magnetic resonance imaging of acute myocardial infarction with and without reperfusion. Am Heart J 1988; 115: 510–8.

24. Caputo GR, Sechtem U, Tscholakoff D, Higgins CB. Measurement of myocardial infarct size at early and late time intervals using MR imaging: An experimental study in dogs. AJR Am J Roentgenol 1987; 149: 237–43.

25. Johnston DL, Homma S, Liu P, Weilbaecher DG, Rokey R, Brady TJ *et al.* Serial changes in nuclear magnetic resonance relaxation times after myocardial infarction in the rabbit: Relationship to water content, severity of ischemia, and histopathology over a six-month period. Magn Reson Med 1988; 8: 363–79.

26. McNamara MT, Higgins CB, Schechtmann N, Botvinick E, Lipton MJ, Chatterjee K *et al.* Detection and characterization of acute myocardial infarction in man with the use of gated magnetic resonance. Circulation 1985; 71: 717–24.

27. Johnston DL, Thompson RC, Liu P, Dinsmore RE, Wismer GL, Saini S *et al.* Magnetic resonance imaging during acute myocardial infarction. Am J Cardiol 1986; 57: 1059–65.

28. Fisher MR, McNamara MT, Higgins CB. Acute myocardial infarction: MR evaluation in 29 patients. AJR Am J Roentgenol 1987; 148: 247–51.

29. Ahmad M, Johnson RF Jr, Fawcett HD, Schreiber MH. Magnetic resonance imaging in patients with unstable angina: Comparison with acute myocardial infarction and normals. Magn Reson Imaging 1988; 6: 527–34.

30. Been M, Smith MA, Ridgeway JP, Brydon JW, Douglas RH, Kean DM, Best JJ *et al.* Characterisation of acute myocardial infarction by gated magnetic resonance imaging. Lancet 1985; 2: 348–50.

31. Been M, Smith MA, Ridgway JP, Douglas RH, De Bono DP, Best JJ *et al.* Serial changes in the T_1 magnetic relaxation parameter after myocardial infarction in man. Br Heart J 1988; 59: 1–8.

32. Postema S, De Roos A, Doornbos J, Krauss XH, Blokland JAK. Recent myocardial infarction: Detection and localization by magnetic resonance imaging and thallium scintigraphy. J Med Imaging 1989; 3: 68–74.

33. Krauss XH, van der Wall EE, Doornbos J, Blokland JAK, Postema S, De Roos A *et al.* The value of magnetic resonance imaging in patients with a recent myocardial infarction: Comparison with planar thallium-201 scintigraphy. Cardiovasc Intervent Radiol 1989; 12: 119–24.

34. Krauss XH, van der Wall EE, Van der Laarse A, Doornbos J, De Roos A, Matheijssen NAA *et al.* Follow-up of regional myocardial T2 relaxation times in patients with myocardial infarction evaluated with magnetic resonance imaging. Eur J Radiol 1990; 11: 110–9.

35. Krauss XH, van der Wall EE, Van der Laarse A, Doornbos J, Matheijssen NAA, De Roos A *et al.* Magnetic resonance imaging of myocardial infarction: Correlation with enzymatic, angiographic, and radionuclide findings. Am Heart J 1991; 122: 1274–83.

36. Filipchuk NG, Peshock RM, Malloy CR, Corbett JR, Rehr RB, Buja LM *et al.* Detection and localization of recent myocardial infarction by magnetic resonance imaging. Am J Cardiol 1986; 58: 214–9.

37. White RD, Cassidy MM, Cheitlin MD, Emilson B, Ports TA, Lim AD *et al.* Segmental evaluation of left ventricular wall motion after myocardial infarction: Magnetic resonance imaging versus echocardiography. Am Heart J 1988; 115: 166–75.

38. White RD, Holt WW, Cheitlin MD, Cassidy MM, Ports TA, Lim AD *et al.* Estimation of the functional and anatomic extent of myocardial infarction using magnetic resonance imaging. Am Heart J 1988; 115: 740–8.

39. Wisenberg G, Finnie KJ, Jablonsky G, Kostuk WJ, Marshall T. Nuclear magnetic resonance and radionuclide angiographic assessment of acute myocardial infarction in a randomized trial of intravenous streptokinase. Am J Cardiol 1988; 62: 1011–6.

40. Johns JA, Leavitt MB, Newell JB, Yasuda T, Leinbach RC, Gold HK *et al.* Quantitation of acute myocardial infarct size by nuclear magnetic resonance imaging. J Am Coll Cardiol 1990; 15: 143–9.

41. Turnbull LW, Ridgway JP, Nicoll JJ, Bell D, Best JJ, Muit AL. Estimating the size of myocardial infarction by magnetic resonance imaging. Br Heart J 1991; 66: 359–63.

42. Brown JJ, Higgins CB. Myocardial paramagnetic contrast agents for MR imaging. AJR Am J Roentgenol 1988; 151: 865–71.

43. Tweedle MF, Eaton SM, Eckelman WC, Gaughan GT, Hagan JJ, Wedeking PW *et al.* Comparative chemical structure and pharmacokinetics of MRI contrast agents. Invest Radiol 1988; 23 (Suppl 1): S236–9.

44. Weinmann HJ, Brasch RC, Press WR, Wesbey GE. Characteristics of gadolinium-DTPA complex: A potential NMR contrast agent. AJR Am J Roentgenol 1984; 142: 619–24.

45. Brasch RC, Weinmann HJ, Wesbey GE. Contrast-enhanced NMR Imaging: Animal studies using gadolinium-DTPA complex. AJR Am J Roentgenol 1984; 142: 625–30.

46. Elster AD, Jackels SC, Allen NS, Marrache RC. Dyke Award. Europeum-DTPA: A gadolinium analogue traceable by fluorescence microscopy. AJNR Am J Neuroradiol 1989; 10: 1137–44.

47. Koenig SH, Spiller M, Brown RD 3d, Wolf GL. Relaxation of water protons in the intra- and extracellular regions of blood containing Gd(DTPA). Magn Reson Med 1986; 3: 791–5.

48. Meyer D, Schaefer M, Bonnemain B. Gd-DOTA, a potential MRI contrast agent. Current status of physicochemical knowledge. Invest Radiol 1988; 23 (Suppl 1): S232–5.

49. Schouman-Claeys E, Frija G, Revel D, Doucet D, Donadieu AM. Canine acute myocardial infarction. *In vivo* detection by MRI with gradient echo technique and contribution of Gd–DOTA. Invest Radiol 1988; 23 (Suppl 1): S254–7.

50. Ogan MD, Schmiedl U, Moseley ME, Grodd W, Paajanen H, Brasch RC. Albumin labeled with Gd-DTPA. An intravascular contrast-enhancing agent for magnetic resonance blood pool imaging: Preparation and characterization. Invest Radiol 1987; 22: 665–71.

51. Schmiedl U, Sievers RE, Brasch RC, Wolfe CL, Chew WM, Ogan MD *et al.* Acute myocardial ischemia and reperfusion: MR imaging with albumin-Gd-DTPA. Radiology 1989; 170: 351–6.

52. Schmiedl U, Ogan M, Paajanen H, Marotti M, Crooks LE, Brito AC *et al.* Albumin labeled with Gd-DTPA as an intravascular, blood pool-enhancing agent for MR imaging: Biodistribution and imaging studies. Radiology 1987; 162: 205–10.

53. Schmiedl U, Ogan MD, Moseley ME, Brasch RC. Comparison of the contrast-enhancing properties of albumin-(Gd-DTPA) and Gd-DTPA at 2.0 T: An experimental study in rats. AJR Am J Roentgenol 1986; 147: 1263–70.

54. Matheijssen NA, De Roos A, van der Wall EE, Doornbos J, Van Dijkman PR, Bruschke AV *et al.* Acute myocardial infarction: Comparison of T2-weighted and T1-weighted gadolinium-DTPA enhanced MR imaging. Magn Reson Med 1991; 17: 460–9.

55. Wesbey GE, Higgins CB, McNamara MT, Engelstad BL, Lipton MJ, Sievers R *et al.* Effect of gadolinium-DTPA on the magnetic relaxation times of normal and infarcted myocardium. Radiology 1984; 153: 165–9.

56. McNamara MT, Higgins CB, Ehman RL, Revel D, Sievers R, Brasch RC. Acute myocardial ischemia: Magnetic resonance contrast enhancement with gadolinium-DTPA. Radiology 1984; 153: 157–63.

57. Runge VM, Clanton JA, Wehr CJ, Partain CL, James AE Jr. Gated magnetic resonance imaging of acute myocardial ischemia in dogs: Application of multi-echo techniques and contrast enhancement with GD DTPA. Magn Reson Imaging 1985; 3: 255–66.

58. Johnston DL, Liu P, Lauffer RB, Newell JB, Wedeen VJ, Rosen BR *et al.* Use of Gadolinium-DTPA as a myocardial perfusion agent: Potential applications and limitations for magnetic resonance imaging. J Nucl Med 1987; 28: 871–7.

59. Nishimura T, Yamada Y, Kozuka T, Nakatani T, Noda H, Takano H. Value and limitation of gadolinium-DTPA contrast enhancement in the early detection of acute canine myocardial infarction. Am J Physiol Imaging 1987; 2: 181–5.

60. Miller DD, Holmvang G, Gill JB, Dragotakes D, Kantor HL, Okada RD *et al.* MRI detection of myocardial perfusion changes by gadolinium-DTPA infusion during dipyridamole hyperemia. Magn Reson Med 1989; 10: 246–55.

61. Tscholakoff D, Higgins CB, Sechtem U, McNamara MT. Occlusive and reperfused myocardial infarcts: Effect of Gd-DTPA on ECG-gated MR imaging. Radiology 1986; 160: 515–9.

62. McNamara MT, Tscholakoff D, Revel D, Soulen R, Schechtmann N, Botvinick E *et al.* Differentiation of reversible and irreversible myocardial injury by MR imaging with and without gadolinium-DTPA. Radiology 1986; 158: 765–9.

63. Peshock RM, Malloy CR, Buja LM, Nunnally RL, Parkey RW, Willerson JT. Magnetic resonance imaging of acute myocardial infarction: Gadolinium diethylenetriamine pentaacetic acid as a marker of reperfusion. Circulation 1986; 74: 1434–40.

64. Wolfe CL, Moseley ME, Wikstrom MG, Sievers RE, Wendland MF, Dupon JW *et al.* Assessment of myocardial salvage after ischemia and reperfusion using magnetic resonance imaging and spectroscopy. Circulation 1989; 80: 969–82.

65. Schaefer S, Malloy CR, Katz J, Parkey RW, Buja LM, Willerson JT *et al.* Gadolinium-DTPA-enhanced nuclear magnetic resonance imaging of reperfused myocardium: Identification of the myocardial bed at risk. J Am Coll Cardiol 1988; 12: 1064–72.

66. Holman ER, Van Dijkman PR, van der Wall EE, Matheijssen NA, Van der Meer P, Van Echteld CJ *et al.* Assessment of myocardial perfusion during ischemia and reperfusion in isolated rat hearts using gadopentetic acid-enhanced magnetic resonance imaging. Coronary Artery Dis 1991; 2: 789–97.

67. Nishimura T, Yamada Y, Hayashi M, Kozuka T, Nakatani T, Noda H *et al.* Determination of infarct size of acute myocardial infarction in dogs by magnetic resonance imaging and gadolinium-DTPA: Comparison with indium-111 antimyosin imaging. Am J Physiol Imaging 1989; 4: 83–8.

68. Van Dijkman PR, Hold KM, Van der Laarse A, Holman ER, Özdemir HI, Van der Nat TH *et al.* Sequential analysis of infarcted and normal myocardium in piglets using *in vivo* gadolinium-enhanced MR images. Magn Reson Imaging 1993; 11: 207–18.

69. Eichstaedt HW, Felix R, Dougherty FC, Langer M, Rutsch W, Schmutzler H. Magnetic

resonance imaging (MRI) in different stages of myocardial infarction using the contrast agent gadolinium-DTPA. Clin Cardiol 1986; 9: 527–35.

70. Nishimura T, Kobayashi H, Ohara Y, Yamada N, Haze K, Takamiya M *et al.* Serial assessment of myocardial infarction by using gated MR Imaging and Gd-DTPA. AJR Am J Roentgenol 1989; 153: 715–20.

71. De Roos A, Doornbos J, van der Wall EE, Van Voorthuisen AE. MR imaging of acute myocardial infarction: Value of Gd-DTPA. AJR Am J Roentgenol 1988; 150: 531–4.

72. van der Wall EE, Doornbos J, Postema S, Van Dijkman PRM, Manger Cats V, De Roos A *et al.* Improved detection of myocardial infarction by Gadolinium-enhanced magnetic resonance imaging [abstract]. Eur Heart J 1988; 9 (Abstract Suppl I): 340.

73. Van Dijkman PR, Doornbos J, De Roos A, Van der Laarse A, Postema S, Matheijssen NA *et al.* Improved detection of acute myocardial infarction by magnetic resonance imaging using Gadolinium-DTPA. Int J Card Imaging 1989; 5: 1–8.

74. Van Dijkman PR, van der Wall EE, Doornbos J, Van der Laarse A, Postema S, De Roos A *et al.* Improved assessment of acute myocardial infarction by magnetic resonance imaging and Gadolinium-DTPA [abstract]. J Am Coll Cardiol 1989; 13 (Suppl A): 49A.

75. Van Dijkman PR, van der Wall EE, De Roos A, Matheijssen NA, Van Rossum AC, Doornbos J *et al.* Acute, subacute, and chronic myocardial infarction: Quantitative analysis of gadolinium-enhanced MR images. Radiology 1991; 180: 147–51.

76. Holman ER, van Jonbergen HP, van Dijkman PR, van der Laarse A, de Roos A, van der Wall EE. Comparison of magnetic resonance imaging studies with enzymatic indexes of myocardial necrosis for quantification of myocardial infarct size. Am J Cardiol 1993; 71: 1036–40.

77. van der Wall EE, Van Dijkman PRM, De Roos A, Doornbos J, Van der Laarse A, Manger Cats V *et al.* Diagnostic significance of gadolinium-DTPA (diethylenetriamine penta-acetic acid) enhanced magnetic resonance imaging in thrombolytic treatment for acute myocardial infarction: Its potential in assessing reperfusion. Br Heart J 1990; 63: 12–7.

78. De Roos A, Van Rossum A, van der Wall E, Postema S, Doornbos J, Matheijssen N *et al.* Reperfused and nonreperfused myocardial infarction: Diagnostic potential of Gd-DTPA-enhanced MR imaging. Radiology 1989; 172: 717–20.

79. De Roos A, Matheijssen NA, Doornbos J, Van Dijkman PR, Van Voorthuisen AE, van der Wall EE. Myocardial infarct size after reperfusion therapy: Assessment with Gd-DTPA-enhanced MR imaging. Radiology 1990; 176: 517–21.

80. Haase A. Snapshot FLASH MRI. Application to T1, T2, and chemical-shift imaging. Magn Reson Med 1990; 13: 77–89.

81. Henrich D, Haase A, Matthaei D. 3D-snapshot flash NMR imaging of the human heart. Magn Reson Imaging 1990; 8: 377–9.

82. Frahm J, Merboldt KD, Bruhn H, Gyngell ML, Hanicke W, Chien D. 0.3-second FLASH MRI of the human heart. Magn Reson Med 1990; 13: 150–7.

83. Atkinson DJ, Burstein D, Edelman RR. First-pass cardiac perfusion: Evaluation with ultrafast MR imaging. Radiology 1990; 174: 757–62.

84. Manning WJ, Atkinson DJ, Grossman W, Paulin S, Edelman RR. First-pass nuclear magnetic resonance imaging studies using gadolinium-DTPA in patients with coronary artery disease. J Am Coll Cardiol 1991; 18: 959–65.

85. Van Rugge FP, Boreel JJ, van der Wall EE, van Dijkman PRM, van der Laarse A, Doornbos J *et al.* Cardiac first-pass and myocardial perfusion in normal subjects assessed by sub-second Gd-DTPA enhanced MR imaging. J Comput Assist Tomogr 1991; 15: 959–65.

86. Van Rugge FP, van der Wall EE, van Dijkman PR, Louwerenburg HW, de Roos A, Bruschke AV. Usefulness of ultrafast magnetic resonance imaging in healed myocardial infarction. Am J Cardiol 1992; 70: 1233–7.

87. Buser PT, Auffermann W, Holt WW, Wagner S, Kircher B, Wolfe C *et al.* Noninvasive evaluation of global left ventricular function with use of cine nuclear magnetic resonance. J Am Coll Cardiol 1989; 13: 1294–300.

88. Pattynama PM, Doornbos J, Hermans J, van der Wall EE, De Roos A. Magnetic resonance

evaluation of regional left ventricular function. Effect of through-plane motion. Invest Radiol 1992; 27: 681–5.

89. Pattynama PM, Lamb HJ, Van der Velde EA, van der Wall EE, De Roos A. Left ventricular measurements with cine and spin-echo MR imaging: A study of reproducibility with variance component analysis. Radiology 1993; 187: 261–8.

90. Sechtem U, Sommerhoff BA, Markiewicz W, White RD, Cheitlin MD, Higgins CB. Regional left ventricular wall thickening by magnetic resonance imaging: Evaluation of normal persons and patients with global and regional dysfunction. Am J Cardiol 1987; 59: 145–51.

91. Pflugfelder PW, Sechtem UP, White RD, Higgins CB. Quantification of regional myocardial function by rapid cine MR imaging. AJR Am J Roentgenol 1988; 150: 523–9.

92. Matheijssen NA, De Roos A, Doornbos J, Reiber JH, Waldman GJ, Van der Wall EE. Left ventricular wall motion analysis in patients with acute myocardial infarction using magnetic resonance imaging. Magn Reson Imaging 1993; 11: 485–92.

93. Pettigrew RI. Dynamic cardiac MR imaging. Techniques and applications. Radiol Clin North Am 1989; 27: 1183–203.

94. Baer FM, Smolarz K, Jungehülsing M, Beckwilm J, Theissen P, Sechtem U *et al.* Chronic myocardial infarction: Assessment of morphology, function, and perfusion by gradient-echo magnetic resonance imaging and ^{99m}Tc-methoxyisobutyl-isonitrile SPECT. Am Heart J 1992; 123: 636–45.

95. Perrone-Filardi P, Bacharach SL, Dilsizian V, Maurea S, Marin-Neto JA, Arrighi JA *et al.* Metabolic evidence of viable myocardium in regions with reduced wall thickness and absent wall thickening in patients with chronic ischemic left ventricular dysfunction. J Am Coll Cardiol 1992; 20: 161–8.

96. Perrone-Filardi P, Bacharach SL, Dilsizian V, Maurea S, Frank JA, Bonow RO. Regional left ventricular wall thickening. Relation to regional uptake of 18-fluorodeoxyglucose and 201-Tl in patients with chronic coronary artery disease and left ventricular dysfunction. Circulation 1992; 86: 1125–37.

97. Pennell DJ, Underwood SR, Manzara CC, Swanton RH, Walker JM, Ell PJ *et al.* Magnetic resonance imaging during dobutamine stress in coronary artery disease. Am J Cardiol 1992; 70: 34–40.

98. Van Rugge FP, van der Wall EE, Bruschke AV. New developments in pharmacologic stress imaging. Am Heart J 1992; 124: 468–85.

99. van Rugge FP, Holman ER, van der Wall EE, de Roos A, van der Laarse A, Bruschke AV. Quantitation of global and regional left ventricular function by cine magnetic resonance imaging during dobutamine stress in normal human subjects. Eur Heart J 1993; 14: 456–63.

100. Van Rugge FP, van der Wall EE, de Roos A, Bruschke AV. Dobutamine stress magnetic resonance imaging for detection of coronary artery disease. J Am Coll Cardiol 1993; 22: 431–9.

101. Van Rugge FP, van der Wall EE, Spanjersberg SJ, de Roos A, Matheijssen NA, Zwinderman AH *et al.* Magnetic resonance imaging during dobutamine stress for detection and localization of coronary artery disease. Quantitative wall motion analysis using a modification of the centerline method. Circulation. (July issue, 1994).

102. Zerhouni EA, Parish DM, Rogers WJ, Yang A, Shapiro EP. Human heart: Tagging with MR imaging-a method for noninvasive assessment of myocardial motion. Radiology 1988; 169: 59–63.

103. Bolster BD Jr, McVeigh ER, Zerhouni EA. Myocardial tagging in polar coordinates with the use of triped tags. Radiology 1990; 177: 769–72.

104. Axel L, Dougherty L. MR imaging of motion with spatial modulation of magnetization. Radiology 1989; 171: 841–5.

105. Mosher TJ, Smith MB. A DANTE tagging sequence for the evaluation of translational sample motion. Magn Reson Med 1990; 15: 334–9.

106. Buchalter MB, Weiss JL, Rogers WJ, Zerhouni EA, Weisfeldt ML, Beyar R *et al.* Noninvasive quantification of left ventricular rotational deformation in normal humans using magnetic resonance imaging myocardial tagging. Circulation 1990; 81: 1236–44.

107. Schaefer S. Clinical nuclear magnetic resonance spectroscopy: Insight into metabolism. Am J Cardiol 1990; 66: 45F-50F.
108. de Roos A, van der Wall EE. Magnetic resonance imaging and spectroscopy of the heart. Curr Opin Cardiol 1991; 6: 946-52.
109. de Roos A, Doornbos J, Luyten PR, Oosterwaal LJ, van der Wall EE, den Hollander JA. Cardiac metabolism in patients with dilated and hypertrophic cardiomyopathy: Assessment with proton decoupled P-31 MR spectroscopy. J Magn Reson Imaging 1992; 2: 711-9.
110. Rehr RB, Tatum JL, Hirsch JI, Quint R, Clarke G. Reperfused-viable and reperfused-infarcted myocardium: Differentiation with *in vivo* P-31 MR spectroscopy. Radiology 1989; 172: 53-8.
111. Jacobus WE, Taylor GJ 4th, Hollis DP, Nunnally RL. Phosphorus nuclear magnetic resonance of perfused working rat hearts. Nature 1977; 265: 756-8.
112. Nunnally RL, Bottomley PA. Assessment of pharmacological treatment of myocardial infarction by phosphorus-31 NMR with surface coils. Science 1981; 211: 177-80.
113. Flaherty JT, Weisfeldt ML, Bulkley BH, Gardner TJ, Gott VL, Jacobus WE. Mechanisms of ischemic myocardial cell damage assessed by phosphorus-31 nuclear magnetic resonance. Circulation 1982; 65: 561-70.
114. Rehr RB, Tatum J, Hirsch J, Wetstein L, Clarke G. Effective separation of normal, acutely ischemic, and reperfused myocardium with P-31 MR spectroscopy. Radiology 1988; 168: 81-9.
115. Bailey IA, Seymour AL. Effects of reperfusion on the P-31 NMR spectrum of ischemic rat hearts. Biochem Soc Trans 1981; 9: 234-6.
116. Bailey IA, Seymour AL, Radda GK. A 31P NMR study of the effects of reflow on the ischaemic rat heart. Biochim Biophys Acta 1981; 637: 1-7.
117. Ichihara K, Abiko Y. Rebound recovery of myocardial creatine phosphate with reperfusion after ischemia. Am Heart J 1984; 108: 1594-7.
118. Wroblewski LC, Aisen AM, Swanson SD, Buda AJ. Evaluation of myocardial viability following ischemic and reperfusion injury using phophorus 31 nuclear magnetic resonance spectroscopy *in vivo*. Am Heart J 1990; 120: 31-9.
119. Rehr RB, Fuhs BE, Lee F, Tatum JL, Hirsch JI, Quint R. Differentiation of reperfused-viable (stunned) from reperfused-infarcted myocardium at 1 to 3 days postreperfusion by *in vivo* phosphorus-31 nuclear magnetic resonance spectroscopy. Am Heart J 1991; 122: 1571-82.
120. Bottomley PA, Herfkens RJ, Smith LS, Bahore TM. Altered phosphate metabolism in myocardial infarction P-31 MR spectroscopy. Radiology 1987; 165: 703-7.
121. Blackledge MJ, Rajagopalan B, Oberhaensli RD, Bolas NM, Styles P, Radda G. Quantitative studies of human cardiac metabolism by 31P rotating-frame NMR. Proc Natl Acad Sci USA 1987; 84: 4283-7.
122. Weiss RG, Bottomley PA, Hardy CJ, Gerstenblith G. Regional myocardial metabolism of high-energy phosphates during isometric exercise in patients with coronary artery disease. N Engl J Med 1990; 323: 1593-600.
123. Bottomley PA, Weiss RG, Hardy CJ, Baumgartner WA. Myocardial high-energy phosphate metabolism and allograft rejection in patients with heart transplants. Radiology 1991; 181: 67-75.
124. Bottomley PA, Hardy CJ, Roemer PB. Phosphate metabolite imaging and concentration measurements in human heart by nuclear magnetic resonance. Magn Reson Med 1990; 14: 425-34.
125. de Roos A, Luyten PR, Doornbos J, van der Laarse A, van der Wall EE. Clinical phosphorus-31 magnetic resonance spectroscopy in cardiomyopathy. In Pohost GM (ed): Cardiovascular Applications of Magnetic Resonance. Mount Kisco, NY: Futura 1993; 363-70.
126. Schaefer S, Gober JR, Schwartz GG, Twieg DB, Weiner MW, Massie B. *In vivo* phosphorus-31 spectroscopic imaging in patients with global myocardial disease. Am J Cardiol 1990; 65: 1154-61.

127. Schaefer S, Gober J, Valenza M, Karczmar GS, Matson GB, Camacho SA *et al.* Nuclear magnetic resonance imaging-guided phosphorus-31 spectroscopy of the human heart. J Am Coll Cardiol 1988; 12: 1449–55.
128. Bottomley PA. Noninvasive study of high-energy phosphate metabolism in human heart by depth-resolved 31P NMR spectroscopy. Science 1985; 229: 769–72.
129. Higgins CB. Success of acute thrombolytic therapy and acute myocardial infarction: What does it demand from cardiac imaging in the 1990s? Radiology 1989; 172: 17–9.

8. Approach to the assessment of myocardial viability in the cardiac catheterization laboratory

MORTON J. KERN & MICHAEL S. FLYNN

Introduction

The extent of viable myocardium after acute coronary artery occlusion is critical to both daily function and long-term outcome in patients with coronary artery disease. In addition to the extent of myocardium at risk, the two main determinates of both infarct size and viable myocardium after coronary artery occlusion are the duration of occlusion and extent of collateralization of blood flow to the occluded vascular bed [1–5]. In the assessment of myocardial viability, techniques within the cardiac catheterization laboratory have been historically the first used and today represent an additional methodology to secure knowledge that revascularization of stunned or hibernating myocardium may provide clinical benefit over the risks involved with coronary revascularization through either surgical or percutaneous angioplasty techniques.

In the assessment of myocardial viability through catheterization laboratory techniques, the assessment of contractile reserve using analysis of left ventricular wall motion has remained a standard examination with regional and global changes from baseline compared to provocative maneuvers (Table 8.1). Although limited in specificity, post-extrasystolic potentiation, exercise, inotropic stimulation and coronary vasodilators have been used to augment regional wall motion asynergy, predicting improvement after revascularization. The non-invasive techniques measuring left ventricular function have generally supplanted left ventriculography with similar data associated with improvement of left ventricular function after revascularization of impaired segments previously demonstrating stimulated improvement [6]. Alterations in regional and global left ventricular function during pacing, vasopressor stimulation and left ventricular hemodynamic responses to ischemia provoking interventions can be assessed in the catheterization laboratory. Myocardial viability is implicated when such interventions alter left ventricular wall motion in an appropriate manner.

Myocardial viability is also related to coronary anatomy. Coronary arteriography permits assessment of blood supply to infarcted but viable myocardial zones. The collateral circulation angiographically can be semi-quantitatively gauged and is a major predictor of myocardial viability. Most recently, a Doppler-tipped angioplasty guidewire technique can now assess both

A.S. Iskandrian and E.E. van der Wall (eds): Myocardial viability, 141–161.
© 1994 *Kluwer Academic Publishers.*

Table 8.1. Approach to the assessment of myocardial viability in the cardiac catheterization laboratory

Left ventriculography
  1. Global ejection fraction
  2. Velocity of circumferential shortening
  3. Regional contractile reserve
     a. Post-extrasystolic potentiation
     b. NTG
     c. Epinephrine or other inotropic agents (Dobutamine)
     d. Isoproterenol
     e. Exercise

Coronary Angiography
  1. Extent and severity of epicardial luminal obstruction
  2. Collateral supply

Hemodynamic alterations during ischemia provoking maneuvers
  1. Pacing
  2. Cold pressor
  3. Inotropic stimulation

the stenosis severity, as well as quantitative grade and direction of collateral flow in regions during diagnostic angiography or coronary angioplasty. The extent of coronary artery disease demonstrated angiographically plays a major role in predicting which myocardial zones may improve after revascularization.

In this chapter we will examine the use of left ventriculography with provocative maneuvers, hemodynamic alterations, and findings on coronary angiography which suggest that tissue viability may be present in asynergic myocardial regions.

Definition of viable myocardium through catheterization laboratory techniques

Viable myocardium is defined as that myocardial tissue which remains potentially responsive in terms of increasing contractile function from a resting hypokinetic or akinetic state after restoration of impaired coronary blood flow [3, 4]. Two conditions of viable myocardial function are thought to exist, hibernating and stunned myocardium. Hibernating myocardium is a state of persistently impaired regional myocardial function at rest due to reduced coronary blood flow. This state can be partially or completely restored to normal if myocardial oxygen supply/demand relationship is improved by restoration of myocardial blood flow or significant reduction in myocardial oxygen demand. In hibernating myocardium, the level of blood flow reduction is generally such that neither myocardial necrosis nor ischemic symptoms occur to indicate potential viability on a clinical basis. Rahimtoola [3] proposed the term 'hibernating myocardium' in 1984 at a National Heart, Lung, and Blood

Institute workshop on the treatment of coronary artery disease where painless ischemia was a widely recognized phenomenon. Improvement of presumed viable myocardial function could be identified through longitudinal studies of coronary artery bypass surgery and left ventricular function re-evaluation.

Stunned myocardium may be distinguished from hibernating myocardium [5]. Stunned myocardium is transient left ventricular dysfunction as a result of stress-induced ischemia, most commonly occurring during acute coronary occlusion of myocardial infarction. Stunned myocardium recovers in association with the restoration of coronary blood flow after complete, or nearly complete, coronary occlusion. Both hibernation and stunning may coexist in the same myocardial bed. In hibernating and stunned myocardium, according to Braunwald and Kloner [5], reduced but sufficient coronary blood flow to impaired myocardium occurs without permanent myocardial dysfunction, or biochemical and ultrasonic abnormalities which may have existed for prolonged periods. In hibernating myocardium, myocardial function remains impaired within the impaired zone supplied by collateral vessels and/or an obstructed or partly obstructed coronary artery. In many patients presenting with akinetic myocardial zones following infarction, coronary blood flow is generally not fully restored, thus the region of impairment can be infarcted, stunned or hibernating or both. These syndromes are physiologically different and are separated by the short-term response to coronary reperfusion. Total occlusion is a requirement of stunned myocardium, demonstrated in experimental animal studies. Therefore, stunned myocardium would be expected to be an association more of acute myocardial infarction, variant angina, and during transient coronary occlusion of interventional procedures, such as angioplasty, whereas hibernating myocardium is apparently associated with more prolonged ischemic insults of a chronic nature in patients with coronary artery disease. Coronary arteriographic findings are important in differentiating these conditions.

Techniques and limitations of ventriculographic analysis

The detection of hibernating or stunned myocardium is poor using subjective or purely clinical evaluations. Ventriculography employs techniques super-imposing end-systolic on end-diastolic contrast-filled contours (Figure 8.1) [7, 8]. Altered alignment of the basal aortic plane can influence assessment of regional wall motion. Regional wall motion improving or deteriorating could thus be erroneously identified if this technique is not precisely performed.

The centerline method of Sheehan *et al.* [9, 10] provides a more reliable and consistent measurement of regional wall motion (Figure 8.2). Changes between the basal and stimulated contractile state can be easily assessed. However, automatic or operator-defined contrast-filled left ventricular contours at the end of each cardiac phase can be the source of additional technical errors. Accurate ventriculography is predicated on satisfactory chamber opacification

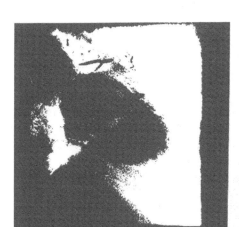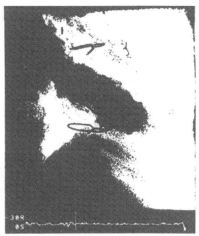

Diastole   Systole

Figure 8.1. Left ventricular contrast angiogram. Superimposition of end-systolic and end-diastolic frames form the basis for left ventricular function analysis.

by performing standardized views (30° RAO) with constant injection rates and having ectopy free periods available for analysis (except when using extrasystolics as the provocative maneuver). Current ventriculographic catheters favor the multi-side holed pigtail configuration as the most reliable to limit ectopy. Future catheter designs may further reduce left ventricular ectopy during contrast injection.

After reperfusion of stunned or hibernating myocardium, viability would more confidently be accepted when global, as well as regional left ventricular systolic function, as reflected by the ejection fraction, were to improve. However, the ejection fraction must, by necessity, be augmented in at least 2 or more myocardial regions to result in an improved global ejection fraction [11].

Limitations of ventriculographic analysis involve the methodology of superimposition of end-diastolic and end-systolic images. There is no existing consensus for selection of fixed reference points for wall motion analysis. Chaitman *et al.* [7] and Leighton *et al.* [8] have proposed methods for selection of fixed reference points, avoiding motion-induced artifact due to respirations altering the long axis of the ventricle and complicating the image placement by systolic movement in an apical direction. Although such factors may not affect the analysis of gross contraction, lesser degrees of wall motion abnormalities, such as hypokinesis, may be over- or under-estimated quantitatively due to the reference point shift. Using the centerline method, these discrepancies may be eliminated.

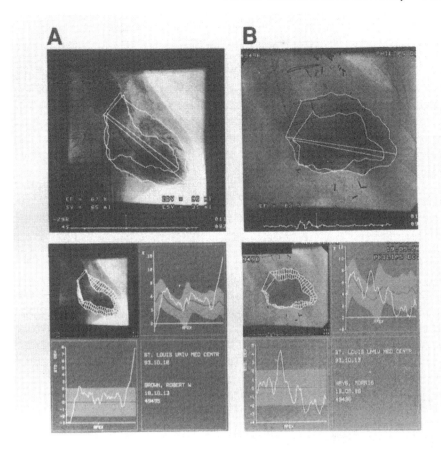

Figure 8.2. A) Centerline method of regional wall motion analysis using the Phillips DCI-ACA program. End-diastolic and end-systolic left ventricular endocardial contours are automatically traced and manually corrected. A centerline is constructed by the computer midway between the two contours. Motion is measured along 100 chords constructed perpendicular to the centerline. Motion at each chord is normalized by the end-diastolic perimeter to yield a shortening fraction. Motion along each chord is plotted for the patient (dark line). The mean motion in the normal ventriculogram group (thin line) and 1 SD above and below the mean (shaded area) are shown for comparison. Wall motion is also plotted as the difference in units of SDs from the normal mean (right panel). The normal ventriculogram group mean is represented by the horizontal zero line. B) Abnormal regional wall motion by centerline method (Courtesy of Phillips, Inc.) Modified with permission [26].

Interventional ventriculography used to assess myocardial viability

Nitroglycerin ventriculography

To assess whether myocardial function can increase in response to improving blood flow, ventriculography during the administration of nitroglycerin has been proposed to identify improvement. Sensitivity, specificity, and accuracy of a nitroglycerin contrast ventriculogram for the detection of hibernating myocardium has been proposed at 76, 65 and 70%, respectively [12]. The improvement in left ventricular wall motion with nitroglycerin is associated with an 85% chance of improvement after bypass surgery.

The technique is straightforward. Left ventriculography is performed prior to and 4–6 minutes after the administration of 0.4 mg sublingual nitroglycerin. In most studies, data were collected in patients after receiving 0.4 to 0.8 mg IV atropine and an IM or IV sedative, such as diazepam (5–10 mg). Quantitative analysis of end-diastolic and end-systolic frames using the apex and mid aortic valve as fixed points for superimposition of the individual angiographic frames. A hypokinetic zone was defined as that which demonstrated < 25% hemi-axis shortening on the initial ventriculogram. An asynergic segment was considered to respond when it normalized or changed to a lesser degree of wall motion abnormality. For example, a dyskinetic segment becoming akinetic or an akinetic segment improving to a hypokinetic wall motion. An asynergic segment was considered improved when it showed a ≥ 10% increase in hemi-axis shortening.

McAnulty *et al.* [12] identified improvement in left ventricular wall motion following nitroglycerin during contrast ventriculography. In 25 patients with resting left ventricular wall motion abnormalities, left ventriculography was performed as described above. Sixteen patients had coronary artery disease, 6 had no coronary artery disease, and 3 had congestive cardiomyopathy with normal coronary arteriography. In 7 of 12 patients with coronary artery disease, abnormal segmental wall motion improved after nitroglycerin. In 5, left ventricular wall motion did not change. Heart rate, left ventricular systolic and end-diastolic pressures, as well as end-diastolic volumes were not different for patients whose wall motion improved compared to those who did not. In patients whose wall motion improved after nitroglycerin, ejection fraction increased from 0.47 to 0.62 (*p* < 0.05). In those without improvement, the ejection fraction remained unchanged at 0.55 to 0.58 ± 0.051 (an insignificant change). Patients with congestive cardiomyopathy showed no improvement after nitroglycerin. The investigators concluded that left ventricular wall motion abnormalities and ejection fraction can be improved in some patients with coronary artery disease following nitroglycerin. The mechanism of effect as this time was unknown.

A similar study was performed by Helfant *et al.* [13] in which improvement in wall motion after nitroglycerin ventriculography to unmask reversible asynergy correlated with post-bypass ventriculographic improvement in wall motion. In left ventricular segments which were responsive to nitroglycerin, coronary artery bypass grafting improved regional synergy. A positive response to nitroglycerin appeared to be predictive of corresponding beneficial effects from coronary revascularization. The investigators suggested that nitroglycerin ventriculography should be used to assess this phenomenon.

Banka *et al.* [14] established the comparative value of nitroglycerin post-extrasystolic potentiation and nitroglycerin plus extra post-systolic potentiation (*vide infra*) for unmasking asynergic residual contractile ability during left ventriculography. In 36 patients undergoing cardiac catheterization for the evaluation of coronary artery disease with asynergy on ventriculography, the relative value of these 3 modalities for the unmasking of asynergic residual contraction was compared. Each patient was used as his own control. Regional asynergy was defined as a localized abnormality of left ventricular contraction. The appearance of 1–3 premature ventricular beats during the contract injection during ventriculography on an initial ventriculogram was required in addition to a post-nitroglycerin ventriculogram. Coronary artery disease of > 75% diameter reduction in 1 or more of 3 vessels and the absence of angiographic evidence of other etiologic heart disease were also inclusion criteria.

The protocol of Banka *et al.* [14] was performed in two parts in which ventricular ectopic beats were present on the initial ventriculogram, but not during the nitroglycerin ventriculogram. Control ventriculography was compared to post-extrasystolic beat potentiation (post-extrasystolic potentiation) and nitroglycerin ventriculography. In a subgroup of 13 patients, a nitroglycerin ventriculogram was accompanied by ventricular premature beats allowing comparison between control nitroglycerin and nitroglycerin plus extrasystolic potentiation.

The results of this study indicated that of 15 akinetic zones, 4 improved with both nitroglycerin and post-extrasystolic potentiation (Figure 8.3). Ten zones were unchanged. One akinetic zone improved with nitroglycerin, but remained unchanged with post-extrasystolic potentiation. Four dyskinetic zones did not change with either intervention. Six akinetic zones responding to nitroglycerin alone further improved when nitroglycerin was evaluated with post-extrasystolic potentiation. However, none of the 13 nitroglycerin unresponsive zones had favorable alterations after a combination of nitroglycerin and post-extrasystolic potentiation. These maneuvers each appeared equally capable of unmasking asynergic residual contractility.

Assessment of inotropic contractile reserve with post-extrasystolic potentiation of regional and global asynergy

Additional methods to identify change in ventriculographic wall motion function have included inotropic stimulation and post-extrasystolic potentiation, both of which increase the force of contraction of the normal myocardium and accentuate the tethering effect on an akinetic non-viable

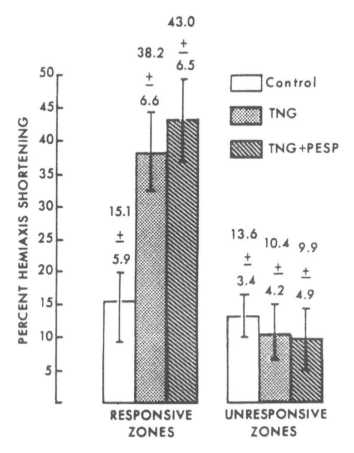

Figure 8.3. Comparative effect of nitroglycerin (TNG) and nitroglycerin plus post-extrasystolic potentiation (TNG + PESP) on asynergic zones. The further change in responsive zones when TNG + PESP was applied was significant (P < 0.001). None of the changes in the unresponsive zones were statistically significant. With permission [14].

segment. These interventions appear to demonstrate an improvement of akinetic wall motion due to hibernating or stunned muscle. Studies demonstrating the improvement of left ventricular segments during inotropic stimulation, however, may not always yield compelling improvement after bypass surgery [15–19].

As an initial physiologic basis for using post-extrasystolic potentiation in the catheterization laboratory, Dyke *et al.* [17, 18] studied latent function in acutely ischemic myocardium in experimental canine models and in patients with coronary artery disease. The use of pharmacologic inotropic stimulation and post-extrasystolic potentiation were also studied in the canine model using controlled reduction of coronary blood flow. Segmental shortening and left ventricular pressure were used to construct left ventricular pressure-length loops identifying functional left ventricular alterations during myocardial ischemia of various regional segments. Acute ischemia depressed segmental function with reduction in regional shortening of $-20 \pm 0.2\%$ with dyskinesia. Restoration of coronary blood flow corrected the abnormal shortening to normal levels. During acute regional ischemia, post-extrasystolic potentiation augmented the regional function $49 \pm 0.3\%$ and eliminated dyskinesia. Isoproterenol or intravenous calcium did not produce comparable changes with only a $9 \pm 0.5\%$ improvement in regional shortening. With pharmacologic stimulation, there was no consistent change in total segment shortening and minimal alterations or reduction in the pressure-length loop in the regionally impaired zone. The investigators concluded that pharmacologic agents accentuated early dyskinesia but caused no consistent improvement in total shortening. Post-extrasystolic potentiation, in contrast to pharmacologic stimulation, either worsened systemic function or caused responses that were minimal and inconsistent. These and other investigators further suggested that these responses cannot be useful to identify ischemic but viable myocardium [17, 18].

In patients, Dyke *et al.* [17] also examined global and segmental wall motion during ventriculography following coronary revascularization identifying the successful reversibility of impaired ischemic left ventricular myocardium in patients with coronary artery disease. The investigators evaluated the effectiveness of post-extrasystolic potentiation to predict latent contractile reserve in this patient group. Quantitative ventriculography in 15 patients with coronary artery disease, 7 with significant asynergistic wall motion abnormalities and 17 controls, was examined at baseline and again after a single extrasystolic beat introduced by an R-wave coupled stimulator. Improved segmental axis shortening was observed in 51 of 55 axes of the ventriculograms. Fifteen of 17 hypokinetic or akinetic axes improved. It was also noted that improvement in both global ejection fraction and mean rate of circumferential fiber shortening occurred in 17 or 18 patients (Figures 8.4, 8.5). No significant arrhythmia was induced with this technique. The use of a single interposed beat with post-extrasystolic potentiation during ventriculography appeared to be a safe and effective method to detect residual contractile dysfunction that may benefit by revascularization.

Post-extrasystolic potentiation appeared to have advantages over pharmacologic inotropic stimulation to detect latent or residual myocardial function in patients with coronary artery disease. Pharmacologic responses may be attenuated or resultant secondary to ischemic depression of myocardial function. Pharmacologic vasodilators may induce coronary steal which may accompany beta-mediated vasodilatation with isoproterenol resulting in further ischemic and contractile depression of endomyocardial layers while global ventricular function demonstrated an improvement [18–21]. One important aspect in human subjects is that pharmacologic inotropic stimulation necessitates two ventriculograms, a technical inconvenience which may unnecessarily prolong studies in critically ill individuals who may have the most myocardium at risk in which viability needs to be determined. Post-extrasystolic

150   *M.J. Kern & M.S. Flynn*

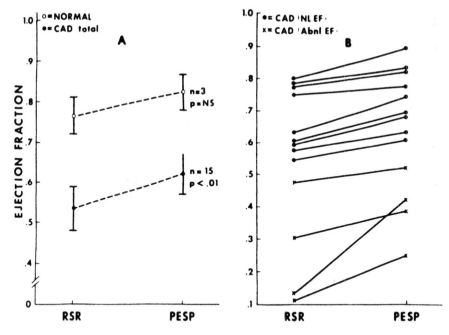

Figure 8.4. A) Effect of post-extra systolic potentiation (PESP) on ejection fraction (EF) in normal controls and patients with coronary artery disease (CAD). B) responses of individual CAD patients with normal and abnormal EF. Vertical bars = mean ± SEM. Wit permission [18].

potentiation is a fundamental and characteristic response of normal cardiac muscle. In the acutely ischemic but viable myocardium, post extrasystolic potentiation may restore normal function prior to re-establishment of coronary blood flow. An ischemic zone rendered hypo- or asynergistic will increase to normal or hypokinetic, respectively. In experimental animal preparations [18], a comparison of pharmacologic stimulation to post-extrasystolic potentiation showed that post-extrasystolic potentiation consistently demonstrated muscle viability with improved segmental and overall ventricular performance through normalization of the segmental shortening pattern in the ischemic zone, while pharmacologic stimulations produced responses which were minimal and highly variable. In canine or human studies, post-extrasystolic potentiation is safe with no adverse effects on ventricular rhythm and required a very simplified methodology. Post-extrasystolic potentiation was easily performed within the cardiac catheterization laboratory.

Nesto *et al.* [22] examined the change in ejection fraction of 10% or more after post-extrasystolic potentiation or epinephrine infusion to discriminate short-term prognosis for medically or surgically treated coronary artery disease with left ventricular wall motion abnormalities. The study related inotropic contractile reserve to 5-years prognosis in 54 patients from 1971 to 1974. Five-year survival was significantly better in patients whose ejection fraction changed > 10% in both the surgically treated group (16 of 20 patients vs 5 of 15 patients)

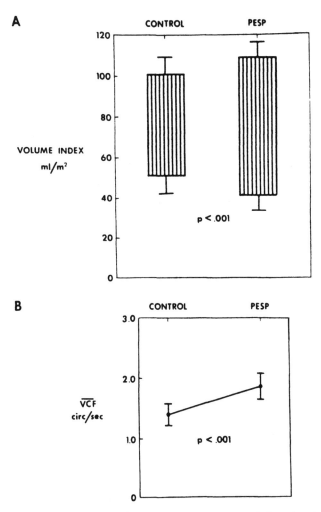

Figure 8.5. A) Effect of post-extra systolic potentiation (PESP) on end-diastolic volume index and end-systolic volume index and B) mean rate of circumferential fiber shortening (VCF in circumferences per second). With permission [18].

and in the medically treated group (6 of 8 patients vs 1 of 11 patients). Among the surviving patients in the surgical group the ejection fraction by radionuclide ventriculography on follow-up was significantly greater in those who demonstrated inotropic contractile reserve in the cardiac catheterization laboratory by contrast ventriculography. The response of inotropic stimuli on reversible wall motion abnormalities appears similar to that seen with nitroglycerin and is associated with a prognosis after bypass surgery which is improved at both 1 and 5 years [11, 22]. These findings were among the strongest data supporting the concept that coronary revascularization can enhance the function of ischemic impaired but viable myocardium. The mechanism of post-extrasystolic potentiation involves not only augmentation of the end-diastolic volume due to the prolonged RR cycle length of compensatory filling, but also related to calcium flux through release of intramyocardial ion stores during the post-extrasystolic beat [20].

Mechanisms of post-extrasystolic potentiation on left ventricular function

The mechanisms involved in augmenting wall motion abnormalities thought to be due to hibernating or stunned myocardium with nitroglycerin or post-extrasystolic potentiation are complex. Several hemodynamic changes occurring in the ventricle with these maneuvers may be responsible for bringing about the enhanced contraction observed in the study of Banka *et al.* [14] and others [17, 18, 21, 23]. Extrasystolic potentiation is associated with a pause, prolonged left ventricular filling and an elevation of the left ventricular end-diastolic pressure with a fall in aortic pressure resulting in decreased initial outflow resistance or afterload. Both mechanisms act to increase myocardial contractility would thus enhance contraction of a potentially viable zone with impaired basal wall motion. The mechanism of nitroglycerin is postulated to occur due to a decrease of afterload and preload with a subsequent minimal increase in heart rate more than mere coronary flow augmentation. Nitroglycerin would thus improve the balance between myocardial oxygen supply and demand favoring enhanced contraction in the asynergic zone due to ischemia. Although the two mechanisms postulated are different, the responses of both interventions within the asynergic zone and left ventricle as a whole are similar. Banka *et al.* [14] noted that the combined effect of nitroglycerin and post-extrasystolic potentiation unmasked residual contractility in asynergic zones not responsive to either intervention alone.

The epinephrine ventriculogram

The augmentation of left ventricular contraction pattern in coronary artery disease by intravenous infusion of inotropic catecholamines such as epinephrine has been associated with identification of ischemic but viable myocardium. Horn *et al.* [24] assessed the potential improvement in abnormal left ventricular wall motion in 18 subjects, 16 with coronary artery disease and left ventricular asynergy by cardiac catheterization and cine ventriculography. Ventriculography was performed at rest and during constant infusion of epinephrine at 1–4 μg/minute after 9 minutes of steady state [25]. The epinephrine infusion induced augmentation of left ventricular contraction in both normal subjects and in all normal zones in the 16 subjects with asynergy, and in no instance was contraction in a normal zone rendered abnormal. Eleven of 16 patients demonstrated improvement in asynergistic regions, 2 of which were previously paradoxic in motion. Of 44 asynergic zones, 23 demonstrated improved contraction during epinephrine ventriculography. One showed depressed contraction. Two had both an increase and deterioration in the same zone of which there were paradoxically moving. Eighteen had no change. Heart rate, left ventricular systolic pressure, left ventricular end-diastolic pressure were slightly increased with epinephrine but not significantly changed from control values. Epinephrine resulted in an increase in both stroke volume and ejection fraction. In 4 subjects who underwent aneurysmectomy, pre-operative lack of improvement with epinephrine ventriculography correlated with pathologic myocardial fibrosis. Epinephrine provoked no adverse reactions, arrhythmias or complications beside brief angina pectoris in 2 subjects. The investigators concluded that left ventricular wall motion abnormalities could be improved or changed in certain cases by inotropic stimulus using epinephrine suggesting residual contractile reserve and that this function differentiates between viable and non-viable zones of functioning myocardium.

The mechanism to augment contraction using epinephrine, and likely other positive inotropic agents, is thought to be an increase in cardiac output, stroke volume, systolic ejection rate without a significant change in blood pressure or heart rate, and act as a secondary coronary vasodilator increasing coronary blood flow [24]. The use of epinephrine was thought to be safer than norepinephrine or isoproterenol in patients with coronary artery disease due to the primary vasoconstrictor effects of norepinephrine and the chronotropic and peripheral vasodilating effects of the beta agonist isoproterenol. These studies were performed using ionic, high osmolar contrast media which was associated with transient myocardial dysfunction due to hypervolemia, myocardial depression and elevation of left ventricular end-diastolic pressure that has been reported with this early type of cardiac radiographic contrast media.

Limitations of post-extrasystolic potentiation as a predictor of potential myocardial viability

Popio *et al* [15] attempted to predict reversibility of ventricular dysfunction prior to coronary artery bypass surgery with post-extrasystolic potentiation. Left ventricular wall motion was studies using traditional cine ventriculography in 31 patients before and after coronary bypass surgery. The pre-operative ejection fraction and wall motion were analyzed in sinus rhythm and again after a random ventricular extra systole. Post-operative ejection fraction and wall motion were examined only during sinus beats. In general, the improvement in global ventricular wall motion correlated with changed in vascular supply provided by revascularization (Figure 8.6). Six of 7 patients whose ejection fraction increased post-operatively had shown post-extrasystolic potentiation. This finding was compared to that of only 10 of 24 patients without such improvement. Regional wall motion improvement also showed a significant association between post-extrasystolic potentiation and post-operative recovery. Of 26 zones successfully revascularized, 11 showed increased wall motion post-operatively. All 11 had post-extrasystolic potentiation compared

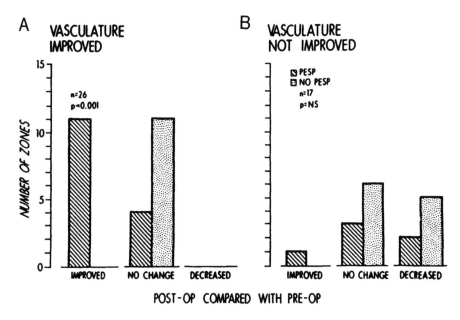

Figure 8.6. Comparison of the occurrence of pre-operative (PRE-OP) regional post-extrasystolic potentiation (PESP) in zones classified on the basis of post-operative (POST-OP) regional motion. A) Only zones judged to have operative improvement in vasculature. B) Zones without operative improvement. Fisher exact test analysis. n = number of patients; NS = not significant; p = probability. With permission [15].

to only 5 of 15 zones without post-operative wall motion increase who demonstrated no post-extrasystolic potentiation. The investigators concluded that post-extrasystolic potentiation appeared to be useful as a predictor of asynergic myocardium improvement following coronary revascularization. However, the technique has a wide range of responses. Those patients with post-extrasystolic potentiation appeared to respond significantly more favorable than those without post-extrasystolic potentiation (Figure 8.7). The limited specificity of this test resulted in failure of this method to be incorporated into routine clinical practice within the cardiac catheterization laboratory. Previous studies [7, 8, 11, 14, 17, 22] showed potentiation in most subjects did not take into account the interobserver variation in the calculation of ejection fraction, which may be as great as 0.1 with an average of 0.5 units. Nonetheless, the degree of augmentation of contraction appeared valuable in separating potentially reversible ischemic zones from non-viable zones. The percent change in ejection fraction using the post-extrasystolic potentiation technique should exceed 0.1 and a > 10% hemiaxis shortening to avoid intraobserver technical error.

The use of the ejection fraction is an easy and universally accepted measure of left ventricular function. However, the separate behavior of zones of myocardium which may improve following revascularization will depend on regional ischemic resolution. In 6 of 10 patients in the study by Popio *et al.* [15]

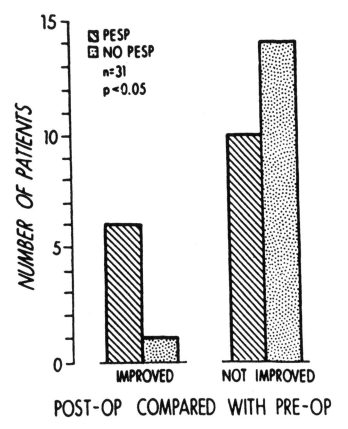

Figure 8.7. Comparison of the occurrence of pre-operative (PRE-OP) post-extrasystolic potentiation (PESP) of the ejection fraction in ventricles with and without post-operative (POST-OP) improvement of the ejection fraction. Chi-square analysis. n = number of patients; p = probability. With permission [15].

with both pre-operative potentiation of the ejection fraction and successful revascularization, improvement in the post-operative ejection fraction occurred in only 1 of 5 who had successful revascularization without pre-operative extrasystolic potentiation. Thus, the overall ejection fraction may not reflect improvement in myocardial viability using a global figure. Despite these significant limitations, pre-operative post-extrasystolic potentiation of the global ejection fraction was associated with post-operative improvement after revascularization. When patients were subgrouped on the basis of the degree of surgical revascularization, the ejection fraction was not a significant factor predicting myocardial viability.

Although this study [15] was heralded as one of the first clinical links between myocardial viability and ventriculographic responses, the limitations of the study design(s) are worth noting. First, there were relatively few patients fulfilling the criteria for inclusion in the retrospective study of Popio *et al.* [15]. The timing of ventricular premature beats may be of concern in which a correlation between the length of the RR coupling interval to the ventricular premature beat has the ability to augment contraction of the premature ventricular contraction beat to a different degree. Popio *et al.* [15] used ventricular premature beats which were spontaneous and showed considerable variation in timing. Late ventricular beats might not be associated with potentiation in certain areas that might improve with a potentiated beat and shorter RR coupling interval. The variability in timing of premature beats must be considered a significant source of error for the post-extrasystolic potentiation evaluation.

In addition to cycle length and augmented post-extrasystolic potentiation/ contractility, there are a large number of variables affecting systolic performance of the left ventricle, particularly when assessing pre- and post-operative studies. Factors which improve left ventricular ejection fraction and wall motion in the post-operative state may not have been present pre-operatively and improved left ventricular function may not be due to the results of revascularization alone. Such conditions may include alterations in heart rate, aortic pressure, preload, afterload, mitral regurgitation severity and neurohumoral factors involving contractility independent of those related to restoration of impaired myocardial blood flow.

Finally, technical features of contrast cineangiography using a limited single plane right anterior oblique projection may not permit an adequate approach to those with regions of asynergy which may be obscured by this examination. Special views (LAO cranial) may be required for septal and lateral wall determinations [26].

Role of coronary angiography in assessment of myocardial viability

Coronary artery stenosis plays a large role in predicting whether regional myocardial function can be restored after revascularization. In patients with an unknown etiology of heart failure, hibernating or stunned myocardium is always a consideration. Coronary arteriography is required to establish the extent and severity of atherosclerotic epicardial obstructions. A previous history of myocardial infarction, especially with regional ventricular dysfunction and absence of pathologic Q-waves and a normal R-wave progression across the precordium [3, 4] has a high likelihood of responding to revascularization. Risk factors for coronary atherosclerosis in such patients also suggest potential viable myocardium and confirmation requires data obtained with coronary arteriography. When supplied by a stenosis > 75% narrowing, a region of potential hibernating myocardium can be strongly considered. Coronary artery stenosis > 90%, totally occluded, or filled via collaterals appears to have even a greater potential for supplying hibernating myocardium beyond that of lesser degrees of coronary narrowing [3, 4]. The presence of stress-induced ischemia as manifested through any of the in-laboratory exercise testing modalities coupled with coronary lesions also strongly supports a diagnosis of hibernating or stunned myocardium. This technique applies more to hypokinetic than akinetic segments and evidence for improved function as well as deterioration with ischemic provocation should be sought.

Collateral supply and myocardial viability

Many studies have identified myocardial regions supplied by total coronary occlusions with collateral vessels, both angiographically and lately on contrast echo [27–29] that appear to be able to retain function and are associated with improved viability [29]. There is a strong association between collateral blood flow and myocardial viability in patients with recent myocardial infarction as demonstrated by Sabia *et al.* [29] and others [27, 28]. The successful reperfusion of an occluded infarct-related coronary artery late after myocardial infarction may also result in improved regional wall motion, dependent on whether collateral flow exists to the bed in question. To demonstrate the role of collaterals on myocardial viability, Sabia *et al.* [29] measured regional wall motion by two-dimensional echocardiography at baseline and one month after angioplasty in 43 patients who had myocardial infarction 2–5 weeks prior to the study. The infarct-related artery was totally occluded. The percentage of infarct bed perfused by collateral flow was assessed by using myocardial contrast echocardiography [30]. Twenty-five of 32 patients who had abnormal wall motion at baseline and underwent successful angioplasty improved as compared to only 1 of 9 patients in whom angioplasty was unsuccessful. The percent of infarct bed supplied by collateral flow prior to angioplasty was directly correlated with wall motion and inversely correlated with the wall motion score one month after revascularization. Twenty-three patients in whom > 50% of the infarct bed was supplied by collateral flow had improved wall motion and greater improvement in wall motion one month after the procedure than in 9 patients who had < 50% of the infarct bed supplied by collateral flow. The improvement in left ventricular function was not influenced by the length of time between the infarction and the attempted revascularization procedure. These investigators concluded that myocardium remains viable for prolonged periods in many patients with acute infarction and that an occluded infarct-related artery supplied by collaterals is associated with viability of the tissue in the infarct bed. Coronary angiography can identify collateral flow, however, the grade of collateral flow may not be correlated with absolute terms with the degree of volumetric flow to that region.

In a study by Rentrop *et al.* [31] those patients with > 50% of the myocardial bed supplied by collaterals had a dramatic improvement in left ventricular function during late reperfusion 1 day to 5 weeks after thrombolytic therapy. In contrast, patients with < 50% of the myocardial bed supplied by collaterals had only a very modest left ventricular functional improvement. The importance of collateral and reperfusion combined to achieve viable myocardium was thus demonstrated through angiography after thrombolytic therapy.

Relative myocardial viability patients who demonstrated restoration of left ventricular function after total coronary occlusions supplied by collaterals had correlative findings with thallium imaging [32]. Those patients without viability had lower collateral scores and poor thallium reversibility in the segment under consideration. Collateral blood flow limits myocardial infarct size, permits improvement in myocardial function after myocardial infarction, prevents aneurysm formation and maintains myocardial viability.

Hemodynamic responses in the catheterization laboratory

The role of hemodynamics in assessment of myocardial viability may be related to the genesis of myocardial ischemia due to rapid ventricular pacing, inotropic responses to dobutamine and wall motion abnormalities as put forth in the ventriculography studies and the blood pressure and cardiac output responses to such interventions (Table 8.2 and 8.3). However, there are no direct studies linking the improvement in hemodynamics to absolute improvement in wall motion after coronary revascularization. However, provocative maneuvers inducing ischemic regional left ventricular dysfunction would suggest that hypokinetic or akinetic zones which deteriorate do so because of satisfactory oxygen supply/demand at rest, but the viable portions of muscle become more asynergic during ischemia. Infarcted or chronically scarred myocardium will generally remain unaffected by further ischemic stimulation. Unfortunately, most hemodynamic indexes of left ventricular function are not able to selectively identify regional changes and, thus, are not specific markers for viability. The assessment of viability remains principally in the purview of angiographic and ventriculographic techniques for studies involving the cardiac catheterization laboratory.

Table 8.2. Research techniques to assess ventricular function

Objective	Method
Systolic function	Ventricular pressure-volume (P-V) relationship (simultaneous LV pressure with LV volume by echocardiogram, contrast angiogram, nuclear angiogram or impedance catheter)
	Variables derived: end-systolic P-V slope, intercept; contractility (+dP/dt)
Diastolic function	Ventricular pressure-volume relationship (as above)
	Variables derived: end-diastolic P-V slope, intercept;relaxation (-dP/dt, Tau, K)

Modified with permission from Kern MJ: *The Cardiac Catheterization Handbook*, p. 316.

Table 8.3. Additional research techniques in the catheterization laboratory

LV function	Methods

Pressure-volume relationships
  End systole
  End diastole
	High fidelity pressure
	  LV volume
	  V-gram (cineangiographic, digital)
	  RV-gram
	  Two-dimensional echocardiogram
	  Impedance catheter

Wall stress LV mass Diastolic function	Quantitative ventriculography High fidelity pressure Doppler mitral inflow
Ventricular interaction Aortic impedance	RV/LV high-fidelity pressures Aortic flow velocity, high-fidelity pressure
Ischemia Testing	
Induced tachycardia Isoproterenol, dopamine Transient coronary occlusion	Electrical pacing Pharmacologic infusion Coronary angioplasty

Modified with permission from Kern MJ: *The Cardiac Catheterization Handbook*, p. 317

Acknowledgements

The authors wish to thank the J.G. Mudd Cardiac Catheterization Laboratory Team and Donna Sander for manuscript preparation.

References

1. Schaper W, Frenzel H, Hort W. Experimental coronary artery occlusion. I. Measurement of infarct size. Basic Res Cardiol 1979; 74: 46–53.
2. Reimer KA, Jennings RB. The 'wavefront phenomenon' of myocardial ischemic cell death. II. Transmural progression of necrosis within the framework of ischemic bed size (myocardial at risk) and collateral flow. Lab Invest 1979; 40: 633–44.
3. Rahimtoola SH. The hibernating myocardium. Am Heart J 1989; 117: 211–21.
4. Braunwald E, Rutherford JD. Reversible ischemic left ventricular dysfunction: Evidence for the 'hibernating myocardium'. J Am Coll Cardiol 1986; 8: 1467–70.
5. Braunwald E, Kloner RA. The stunned myocardium: Prolonged, postischemic ventricular dysfunction. Circulation 1982; 66: 1146–9.
6. Smart SC, Sawada S, Ryan T, Segar D, Atherton L, Berkovitz K *et al.* Low-dose dobutamine echocardiography detects reversible dysfunction after thrombolytic therapy of acute myocardial infarction. Circulation 1993; 88: 405–15.
7. Chaitman BR, Bristow JD, Rahimtoola SH. Left ventricular wall motion assessed by using fixed external reference systems. Circulation 1973; 48: 1043–54.

8. Leighton RF, Wilt SM, Lewis RP. Detection of hypokinesis by a quantitative analysis of left ventricular cineangiograms. Circulation 1974; 50: 121–7.

9. Sheehan FH, Bolson EL, Dodge HT, Mathey DG, Schofer J, Woo HW. Advantages and applications of the centerline method for characterizing regional ventricular function. Circulation 1986; 74: 293–305.

10. Chaitman BR, DeMots H, Bristow JD, Rösch J, Rahimtoola SH. Objective and subjective analysis of left ventricular angiograms. Circulation 1975; 52: 420–5.

11. Cohn PF, Gorlin R, Herman MV, Sonnenblick EH, Horn HR, Cohn LH *et al.* Relation between contractile reserve and prognosis in patients with coronary artery disease and a depressed ejection fraction. Circulation 1975; 51: 414–20.

12. McAnulty JH, Hattenhauer MT, Rösch J, Kloster FE, Rahimtoola SH. Improvement in left ventricular wall motion following nitroglycerin. Circulation 1975; 51: 140–5.

13. Helfant RH, Pine R, Meister SG, Feldman MS, Trout RG, Banka VS. Nitroglycerin to unmask reversible asynergy. Correlation with post coronary bypass ventriculography. Circulation 1974; 50: 108–13.

14. Banka VS, Bodenheimer MM, Shah R, Helfant RH. Intervention ventriculography. Comparative value of nitroglycerin, post-extrasystolic potentiation and nitroglycerin plus post-extrasystolic potentiation. Circulation 1976; 53: 632–7.

15. Popio KA, Gorlin R, Bechtel D, Levine A. Postextrasystolic potentiation as a predictor of potential myocardial viability: preoperative analyses compared with studies after coronary bypass surgery. Am J Cardiol 1977; 39: 944–53.

16. Chatterjee K, Swan HJ, Parmley WW, Sustaita H, Marcus H, Matloff J. Depression of left ventricular function due to acute myocardial ischemia and its reversal following aortocoronary saphenous-vein bypass. N Engl J Med 1972; 286: 1117–22.

17. Dyke SH, Cohn PF, Gorlin R, Sonnenblick EH. Detection of residual myocardial function in coronary artery disease using post-extra systolic potentiation. Circulation 1974; 50: 694–9.

18. Dyke SH, Urschel CW, Sonnenblick EH, Gorlin R, Cohn PF. Detection of latent function in acutely ischemic myocardium in the dog: Comparison of pharmacologic inotropic stimulation and postextrasystolic potentiation. Circ Res 1975; 36: 490–7.

19. Dyke SH, Kirk ES, Sonnenblick EH. Heterogeneous transmyocardial function in ischemia [abstract]. Clin Res 1972; 20: 370.

20. Massie BM, Botvinick EH, Brundage BH, Greenberg B, Shames D, Gelberg H. Relationship of regional myocardial perfusion to segmental wall motion: A physiologic basis for understanding the presence and reversibility of asynergy. Circulation 1978; 58: 1154–63.

21. Yue DT, Burkhoff D, Franz MR, Hunter WC, Sagawa K. Postextrasystolic potentiation of the isolated canine left ventricle. Relationship to mechanical restitution. Circ Res 1985; 56: 340–50.

22. Nesto RW, Cohn LH, Collins JJ Jr, Wynne J, Holman L, Cohn PF. Inotropic contractile reserve: A useful predictor of increased 5 year survival and improved postoperative left ventricular function in patients with coronary artery disease and reduced ejection fraction. Am J Cardiol 1982; 50: 39–44.

23. Klausner SC, Ratshin RA, Tybert JV, Lappin HA, Chatterjee K, Parmley WW. The similarity of changes in segmental contraction patterns induced by postextrasystolic potentiation and nitroglycerin. Circulation 1976; 54: 615–23.

24. Horn HR, Telchholz LE, Cohn PF, Herman MV, Gorlin R. Augmentation of left ventricular contraction pattern in coronary artery disease by an inotropic catecholamine. The epinephrine ventriculogram. Circulation 1974; 49: 1063–71.

25. Sullivan JM, Gorlin R. Effect of l-epinephrine on the coronary circulation in human subjects with and without coronary artery disease. Circ Res 1967; 21: 919–23.

26. Deligonul U, Kern MJ, Serota H, Roth R. Angiographic data. In Kern MJ (ed): The Cardiac Catheterization Handbook. St. Louis, MO: Mosby-Year Book 1991: 242–55.

27. Cohen MV. Coronary Collaterals: Clinical and Experimental Observations. Mount Kisco, NY: Futura 1985: 93–185.

28. Schaper W. Collateral pressure-flow relationships in acute and chronic artery occlusion. In Schaper W (ed): The Collateral Circulation of the Heart. Amsterdam: Elsevier 1971: 155–79.

29. Sabia PJ, Powers ER, Ragosta M, Sarembock IJ, Burwell LR, Kaul S. As association between collateral blood flow and myocardial viability in patients with recent myocardial infarction. N Engl J Med 1992; 327: 1825–31.
30. Kaul S, Kelly P, Oliner JD, Glasheen WP, Keller MW, Watson DD. Assessment of regional myocardial blood flow with myocardial contrast two-dimensional echocardiography. J Am Coll Cardiol 1989; 13: 468–82.
31. Rentrop KP, Feit F, Sherman W, Stecy P, Hosat S, Cohen M *et al.* Late thrombolytic therapy preserves left ventricular function in patients with collateralized total coronary occlusion: Primary end point findings of the Second Mount Sinai-New York University Reperfusion Trial. J Am Coll Cardiol 1989; 14: 58–64.
32. Gohlke H, Heim E, Roskamm H. Prognostic importance of collateral flow and residual coronary stenosis of the myocardial infarct artery after anterior wall Q-wave acute myocardial infarction. Am J Cardiol 1992; 67: 1165–9.

9. The cardiac surgeon's viewpoint of myocardial viability

EDNA H.G. VENNEKER, BERTHE L.F. VAN ECK-SMIT &
GERDA L. VAN RIJK-ZWIKKER

Introduction

In 1968, Favaloro introduced coronary artery bypass grafting (CABG) as therapy for coronary artery stenosis [1]. Coronary bypass surgery has evolved since then and is today an important therapeutic option besides percutaneous transluminal angioplasty (PTCA) and conservative treatment for patients with coronary artery disease. Since the introduction of bypass surgery, the indications have been extensively studied to define those patients who may benefit most from this intervention and to identify patients with high risk. In patients with diminished ejection fraction, left main disease, severe two- or three-vessel disease or proximal left anterior descending (LAD) stenosis, or for patients with unstable or, in contrast, mild angina, long-term survival improves and anginal complaints are relieved following bypass surgery [2,3]. Besides symptomatic relief, long-term survival related to the preservation of left ventricular function is an important goal.

Until recently, severe hypokinesis or akinesis of the left ventricular wall was thought to be caused by cell necrosis and subsequent scar formation. However, pharmacological or post-exercise restoration of perfusion may cause significant improvement in regional function in some of these patients [4,5].

The state of reduced blood flow with chronically impaired left ventricular function, which only improves when coronary blood flow is restored, has been referred to as 'hibernating myocardium' [6,7]. Several studies have emphasized that left ventricular ejection fraction may improve following coronary revascularization, especially in patients with impaired left ventricular function [8–10]. However, this group is also at high risk for events following cardiac surgery. Therefore, in patients with impaired left ventricular function, the distinction between viable and nonviable myocardium has become increasingly important, since regional function may improve in viable myocardium following coronary revascularization. Recent studies have revealed that viable myocardial tissue may still be present in areas which sustained a previous myocardial infarction [11,12]. In addition, these segments may also improve in contractile function following revascularization and, therefore, global left ventricular function may improve [13]. Since left ventricular function is closely related to mortality, long-term survival may increase in this group of patients following coronary revascularization [14].

A.S. Iskandrian and E.E. van der Wall (eds): Myocardial viability, 163–178.
© 1994 *Kluwer Academic Publishers.*

Numerous studies have reported the ability of thallium scintigraphy and positron emission tomography (PET) using ^{18}F-fluorodeoxyglucose (FDG) to predict functional recovery following CABG. Also, several studies have investigated the use of thallium scintigraphy for the assessment of graft patency after coronary surgery. In this chapter we review the literature regarding the value of assessment of myocardial viability by thallium-201 scintigraphy, and by PET in predicting the outcome of CABG. Secondly, the predictive value of post-operative thallium scintigraphy for evaluation of graft patency is discussed and, finally, the usefulness of these techniques for patient management from the cardiac surgeon's point of view is discussed.

Complications and survival in coronary artery surgery

The outcome of coronary artery bypass surgery depends on several factors. The first major factor is peri-operative mortality in relation to complications. Peri-operative complications and mortality increase in older patients, in patients with poor left ventricular function, previous coronary revascularization or left main stem disease, and they also depend on the urgency of the operation. Of the 28,528 patients who underwent CABG in Germany in 1991, overall 30-day operative mortality was 2.6% [15]. Christakis *et al.* reported an operative mortality rate of 2.3% in patients with a left ventricular ejection fraction (LVEF) > 40%, 4.8% with an LVEF between 20–40% and 9.8% in patients with an LVEF of <20% [16]. Post-operative complications, such as low-output syndrome, myocardial infarction and morbidity, occurred 2–4 times more often in patients with poor left ventricular function [16]. Several studies have emphasized that the more left ventricular function is impaired, the more patients may benefit from surgical therapy in terms of long-term survival [17–19]. Therefore, in the group of patients with very poor ventricular function (LVEF <20%), it is very important to identify those who may benefit from coronary revascularization instead of undergoing heart transplantation or continuation with medical treatment.

Relief of symptoms and long-term survival are also important components in which early and late graft patency, in addition to progression of coronary sclerosis, plays a crucial role in the outcome of surgery. Several studies have recently been published concerning long-term survival following CABG. The Veterans' Affairs Study Group reported survival rates at one, five, eleven and fifteen years after CABG for patients operated between 1974 and 1979, of 97%, 84%, 56% and 32%, respectively [20].

One other factor which influences survival is incomplete revascularization. Data from the Coronary Artery Surgery Study (CASS) reveal that, in patients with mild and severe angina, cumulative survival was significantly lower in patients with only a single coronary bypass graft, whereas in patients with severe angina, three-vessel disease and diminished left ventricular function, six-year survival was significantly better in those with three or more bypasses [21].

Initially, saphenous veins were used for bypassing stenosed segments of coronary arteries. The patency of saphenous veins is 70% five years after surgery, which decreases to 50–60% after 10 years. In contrast, internal mammary artery (IMA) grafts have a patency rate of about 95% after 10 years [22]. Ten years after IMA grafting of the LAD, mortality and the number of ischemic events in patients is significantly lower, when compared to patients with saphenous vein bypass grafts [22]. Thus, IMA grafts are currently the conduits of choice, irrespective of age or left ventricular function.

Peri-operative and long-term survival in patients with coronary sclerosis has improved because of improved operative techniques. On the other hand, the patient profile has changed over the last decade. The proportion of patients over 70 years of age operated on today is approximately 40% and the number of re-operations has increased to 30% [23]. In addition, the use of thrombolytic agents and PTCA, the development of pharmacologic agents such as ACE inhibitors, and the presence of advanced diabetic arteriosclerosis in the elderly has created a new population of patients with poor ventricular function. This group of high risk patients may outbalance the increased survival rates. In view of the above, assessment of myocardial viability and, especially, the identification of hibernating myocardium may be useful in identifying those patients who might benefit from CABG in terms of preservation of left ventricular function and improved long-term survival. It may also identify those patients who will not benefit enough and who will ultimately die in intensive care after a prolonged period of low cardiac output, criteria which, to date, have not been established.

Pre-operative assessment of myocardial viability

Over the last decade, several techniques based on different characteristics of the myocardium have been investigated to detect myocardial viability. Both thallium scintigraphy, with either planar or single photon emission-computed tomography (SPECT), and PET using FDG are well-accepted methods for the assessment of myocardial viability. However, studies evaluating the predictive value of either technique for functional improvement of viable myocardium were always performed in a small group of patients.

Thallium scintigraphy

Thallium-201 diffuses into the myocardial cell mainly through active transport by the Na-K-ATPase pump. The extraction depends on coronary flow and cell membrane integrity. Because of this latter feature, it is possible to differentiate viable from nonviable myocardium. If the cell membrane is intact, thallium will diffuse into the cell, resulting in normal thallium uptake or complete or partial redistribution on the thallium scintigram. If the cell membrane is not intact, no tracer uptake will occur and a fixed defect will be observed on scintigraphy.

Since the early seventies, myocardial perfusion imaging with thallium-201 has been successfully used to improve detection of coronary stenosis. In combination with an exercise stress test, qualitative analysis of planar thallium perfusion imaging can detect significant coronary artery stenosis (> 50%) with a sensitivity of 91% and a specificity of 86%, whereas quantitative analysis leads to a sensitivity and specificity of 93% and 91%, respectively [24]. When tomographic techniques are used, sensitivity and specificity for detecting coronary artery stenosis of > 50% are 96% and 91%, respectively [25].

The detection of myocardial viability has gained much interest in recent years because of its potential usefulness for patient management. Different protocols for optimal assessment of myocardial viability have been investigated. Stress or rest scintigraphy with early (3–4 hours) or late (8–24 hours) redistribution images have been used to differentiate viable from nonviable myocardium [26–28]. The occurrence of redistribution on early images accurately predicts viable myocardium. In contrast, the absence of redistribution on early images does not necessarily indicate nonviable tissue, since additional ischemia and severe ischemia may also show a lack of redistribution on early images.

Studies using late (8–72 hours) redistribution images have reported that irreversible segments on the early redistribution images fill in after late redistribution [29–31]. Thus, late redistribution is an even more accurate marker of myocardial viability than early redistribution, however, similar to early redistribution, the absence of redistribution is not an accurate predictor of nonviable tissue. It may be possible that defects are invisible after late redistribution due to the loss of imaging quality. Also, since images are acquired on two separate days, it has a disadvantage for the patient.

Recently, reinjection protocols have been investigated to improve detection of viable and nonviable myocardium. Reinjection of thallium, immediately after the 3–4 hour delayed redistibution images, has improved assessment of viable myocardium by 49% of segments which were diagnosed nonviable on the redistribution scintigram [32]. In a study performed at our hospital we found that immediate thallium reinjection after stress imaging, followed by scintigraphy one hour later, may also be superior to stress-redistribution imaging [33]. Although 13% of the persistent defects after stress-reinjection imaging filled in at the redistribution image acquired 3–4 hours later, the occurrence of reverse redistribution of the segments was 15% higher, compared to 1% with the reinjection scintigram.

Several studies have evaluated the ability of thallium-201 scintigraphy to predict functional recovery of segments with reversible defects and the absence of functional improvement of fixed defects after CABG. In these studies, functional recovery is determined by thallium uptake, improvement in wall motion or both. Rozanski *et al.* reported that in 43 segments with reversible defects, improvement in wall motion following coronary bypass surgery was correctly predicted in 35 segments (81%), whereas in 25 of 29 (86%) segments with fixed defects, the inability to improve regional wall motion was correctly predicted [34]. Other studies reported percentages of 57–91% for pre-operatively viable segments to show an improvement in wall motion after

Table 9.1. Thallium-201 to evaluate the functional improvement after CABG

Study	Year	Technique	Pts	Viable with recovery	Nonviable with no recovery
Ritchie [35]	1977	Tl-201 S-RD/R	11/9	5/8 (63%)[a] TU	3/7 (43%)[a] TU
Verani [36]	1978	Tl-201 S	23	45/64 (70%) abnormal segments improved	
Greenberg [37]	1978	Tl-201 S-RD/R	9	6/8 (63%) TU	3/3 (100%) TU
Robinson [38]	1979	Tl-201 S-RD	36	44/61 (72%) TU	1/23 (9%) TU
Hirzel [39]	1980	Tl-201 S-RD	54	31/54 (57%)[a] TU	25/25 (100%)[a] TU
Rozanski [34]	1981	Tl-201 S-RD	25	35/43 (81%) WM	25/29 (86%) WM
Gibson [40]	1983	Tl-201 S-RD	47	83/92 (90%) TU	23/42 (55%) TU
Brundage [41]	1984	Tl-201 S-RD	23	19/29 (66%) WM	NP
Liu [42]	1985	Tl-201 S-RD	52	22/28 (79%) TU	4/16 (25%) TU
Kiat [31]	1988	Tl-201 S-RD	21[b]	67/79 (85%) TU	34/122 (28%) TU
		Tl-201 S-RD 24 h	21[b]	70/74 (95%) TU	30/48 (63%) TU
Tamaki [43]	1989	Tl-201 S-RD	22	15/23 (65%) WM	19/33 (58%) WM
Ohtani [44]	1990	Tl-201 S-RD	24	23/31 (74%) WM	16/30 (53%) WM
				34/43 (79%) TU	15/32 (43%) TU
Ohtani [45]	1991	Tl-201 S-RD	41	67/84 (80%) WM	20/25 (80%) WM
				79/107 (74%) TU	23/26 (89%) TU
Tamaki [46]	1991	Tl-201 S-RD	11	27/31 (87%) WM	12/25 (48%) WM
Contini [47]	1992	Tl-201 S-RD	60	109/125 (87%) TU	62/101 (61%) TU
Berger [48]	1979	Tl-201 R-RD	22	37/48 (77%) TU	5/18 (28%) TU
Iskandrian [49]	1983	Tl-201 R-RD	26	12/14 (86%)[a] WM	7/9 (78%)[a] WM
Mori [50]	1991	Tl-201 R-RD	17	11/14 (79%) WM	23/37 (62%) WM
Naruse [51]	1992	Tl-201 R-RD	42	17/17 (100%) TU	21/32 (66%) TU
Giubbini [52]	1992	Tl-201 R-RD	13	82/100 (82%) WM	14/20 (56%) WM
Ragosta [53]	1993	Tl-201 R-RD	21	81/141 (57%) WM	27/35 (77%) WM
Ohtani [44]	1990	Tl-201 S-RI	24	33/45 (73%) WM	12/16 (75%) WM
				46/58 (79%) TU	14/17 (82%) TU
Tamaki [46]	1991	Tl-201 S-RD-RI	11	38/48 (79%) WM	6/8 (75%) WM
Coleman [54]	1992	Tl-201 S-RI	18[c]	PPV 91% WM	NPV 75% WM
Kuijper [55]	1993	Tl-201 S-RI	26	106/113 (94%) TU	20/30 (67%) TU
Zimmerman [56]	1993	Tl-201 S-RI	36	16/23 (70%) WM	7/8 (88%) WM

NP = not provided; NPV = negative predictive value; PPV = positive predictive value; Pts = patients; R = rest; RD = redistribution; RI = reinjection; S = stress; TU = thallium uptake; WM = wall motion; [a] = pts; [b] = 15 CABG, 6 PTCA; [c] = 12 CABG, 6 PTCA.

revascularization [31,34–56]. The accurate prediction of nonviable tissue with no recovery of wall motion with thallium-201 scintigraphy is between 48% and 88%. The improvement of thallium uptake post-operatively in segments with reversible defects pre-operatively was correctly predicted in 63–100% of the segments. The correct prediction of no improvement in thallium uptake after coronary bypass surgery varied between the different studies and was correctly predicted in 9–100% of the segments. However, despite long-lasting interest in the value of thallium-201 scintigraphy to predict functional outcome following coronary revascularization, no data are available from large multicentre trials. A review of studies concerning thallium-201 for the evaluation and prediction of functional improvement following CABG is given in Table 9.1.

PET using FDG

Another technique for the detection of viable myocardium is the demonstration of metabolic activity in regions with reduced perfusion and dysfunctional ventricular wall motion. The uptake of FDG, a marker of regional exogenous glucose utilization, depends on the dietary state of the patient, cardiac workload, insulin levels, sympathetic drive and, last but not least, the severity of myocardial ischemia. An increase in myocardial FDG uptake in segments with reduced coronary perfusion indicates metabolic active tissue and, therefore, viable myocardium. In 1986, Tillisch et al. studied 17 patients with a diminished left ventricular function prior to and after CABG [57]. They found that 35 of the 41 segments (85%) identified as viable, using FDG PET imaging prior to surgery, had improved regional wall motion following coronary revascularization. Moreover, 24 of 26 (92%) identified as nonviable segments, did not show improvement in wall motion after bypass surgery.

Since then, several studies have been performed to evaluate whether PET FDG is able to accurately predict functional improvement following CABG. Tamaki et al. and Lucignani et al. reported similar values for the prediction of wall motion recovery after coronary revascularization [58,59]. The ability of FDG to predict functional recovery after coronary artery bypass surgery in PET viable segments varies between 52% and 95% in the current available literature, whereas the ability to predict no change in function after coronary revascularization in nonviable segments varies between 59% and 92% [57–65]. This means that 8–41% of the segments identified as nonviable improve in contractile function following revascularization. Since improvement in left ventricular function is closely related to long-term survival, this would mean that the results of coronary revascularization could improve even more if detection of hibernating myocardium improved. An overview of the published studies is listed in Table 9.2.

Table 9.2. PET to evaluate wall motion improvement after CABG

Study	Year	Technique	Pts	Viable with recovery	Nonviable with no recovery
Tillisch [57]	1986	FDG/NH$_3$	17	35/41 (85%)	24/26 (92%)
Schelbert [60]	1987	FDG	17	85%	95%
Tamaki [58]	1989	FDG/NH$_3$	22	18/23 (78%)	18/23 (78%)
Al-Aouar [61]	1990	FDG/NH$_3$	29	PPV 75%	NPV 90%
Tamaki [62]	1991	FDG/NH$_3$	25	21/27 (78%)	21/26 (81%)
Marwick [63]	1992	FDG	23[a]	19/26 (73%)	35/47 (75%)
Lucignani [59]	1992	FDG	14	37/39 (95%)	12/15 (80%)
Tamaki [64]	1993	FDG/NH$_3$	31	23/29 (79%)	43/47 (91%)
Gropler [65]	1993	FDG vs C-11	34[b]	38/73 (52%)	35/43 (81%)

FDG = ^{18}F-deoxyglucose; NPV = negative predictive value; PPV = positive predictive value; pts = patients; [a] = 11 CABG, 12 PTCA; [b] = 24 CABG, 10 PTCA.

In a recently published study, Eitzman *et al.* reported that FDG PET provides good prognostic information in patients with coronary artery disease and diminished left ventricular function [66]. They found that patients with a mismatch on PET imaging, i.e. reduced coronary perfusion with increased metabolic activity, had a significantly higher rate of events if they were not revascularized. The event rate in this group was also significantly higher compared to patients with a match, i.e. decreased blood flow and FDG uptake. Left ventricular function, extent of coronary artery disease and functional class of angina pectoris did not differ between the groups. The authors conclude that FDG PET gives important clinical information concerning these groups of patients. However, this retrospective study was performed in a small group of patients; larger and prospective studies are required to confirm the findings of Eitzman *et al.*

Myocardial viability in relation to the surgical procedure

Given the fact that the morbidity and mortality of patients with normal ventricular function is low and on the order of 2.5–3.5% after CABG [16], our main concern is patients with severely impaired left ventricular function, since patients with risk factors other than cardiac are not included in this chapter. Patients with moderately impaired left ventricular function, an LVEF of 30% or more, and either hypokinetic or akinetic areas comprise one group, while in a second group, patients with ischemic cardiomyopathy and dilated ventricles, the indication for operation, need to be dealt with on a more individual basis. Because complete revascularization has better short-term and long-term results, for the first group, one could postulate that the policy regarding revascularization could be that any vessel graftable on the angiogram will be grafted, regardless whether wall motion is normal or abnormal, without further information on actual myocardial viability of the akinetic areas. Judging from overall mortality rates of less than 5%, and 90% survival rates at 5 years in patients with mild left ventricular dysfunction [3], the aim should be complete revascularization whenever technically possible. The negative effects of additional bypass time and aortic crossclamp time on morbidity and perioperative mortality are not great enough to justify the additional high costs of diagnostic tests. This is supported by the findings in Eitzman's study [66].

In the second group of patients with a dilated ventricle and poor ejection fraction, where akinetic and hypokinetic areas are not easily discerned, the problem is different because these patients have a higher incidence of low cardiac output and arrhythmias after surgery. Part of this patient population will have hibernating myocardial tissue which only after revascularization slowly improves in function. According to the definition of hibernation, these patients cannot be selected by stress echocardiography or dobutamine MRI, where immediate improvement of the wall motion would prove stunning. However, PET scanning and possibly thallium-201 scintigraphy with reinjection may show the perfusion-metabolism mismatch. Because of the slow recuperation of the myocardium after revascularization, these are also the patients who – with the slightest technical problem – will develop a low cardiac output syndrome. Their average stay in the intensive care unit is 12 days in our hospital, not to mention the costs of the low output syndrome treatment. The peri-operative mortality of this group is high, 9.8% and above [16].

The current development of health care budgeting forces us to look again at our operation indications. If we can detect, by careful analysis, which patients may benefit from the operation and which (after some time) will probably die in the intensive care unit, we may be able to use the limited intensive care space and funds more effectively. The total number of surgical procedures, of course, will not be reduced because of the waiting lists for open heart surgery.

Some caution is needed with respect to the data obtained by thallium-201 or PET scanning in patients in whom hibernating myocardium is suspected. For example, patients with a large area of subendocardial infarction, who present a discrete aneurysm or akinetic area on the angiogram, often show a thin epicardial layer of muscle in surgery, while the subendocardium is completely fibrosed. PET scanning certainly will show evidence of viable tissue, and probably thallium-201 as well. But the effect of revascularization of such an area is doubtful because of insufficient flow demand. However, the epicardial muscular layer will prevent further distension of the ventricle and the development of a large aneurysm. Brunken's study on viable myocardium in Q-wave infarction should also be considered in this light [11].

Thus far, we have discussed myocardial viability in patients who are stable. Since both thallium-201 and PET scanning are time-consuming, neither method is applicable for the acute or even semi-acute coronary patient or, for example, the patient with acute complications of a PTCA procedure. In these situations we do not know whether the problem is caused by infarction or by myocardial stunning and we basically have no means to distinguish between the two. In these cases, trans-oesophageal echocardiography (TEE) will tell over time whether wall motion has changed from the original situation and whether it has improved after intervention. TEE, however, is only an indirect indicator of myocardial viability.

Once myocardial viability is established and the decision for surgical intervention has been made, the main purpose of surgery is to restore normal myocardial perfusion and preserve myocardial function. One has to bear in mind, however, that the surgical procedure itself includes a period of complete ischemia in the heart. To minimize the deleterious effects of this ischemic period, the heart (and the patient) is cooled by means of extra-corporal circulation to reduce metabolism. A cardioplegic solution is administered into the coronary arteries to cause cardiac arrest and preserve myocardial energy reserves. If the (viable) myocardium is perfused almost exclusively through collateral circulation, which is often the case in re-operations and left main stem stenosis with occluded right coronary artery, myocardial protection will be less optimal since there will be a delay in the delivery of the cardioplegic solution.

Administering the cardioplegic solution retrogradely into the coronary sinus has solved part of this problem. Yet, it is conceivable, that with delayed cardioplegic arrest and, thus, insufficient myocardial protection, the (hibernating) myocardium may be irreversibly damaged and myocardial infarction will occur irrespective of the presence of a patent graft. In patients with poor left ventricular function, the surgical procedure causes, at best, a transient status of stunning or reperfusion injury; the clinical picture of low cardiac output often improves after 6–8 hours [67]. Consequently, the prediction of viable myocardium does not necessarily predict the clinical outcome of the procedure.

The chronic ischemia which causes the myocardium to hibernate may also damage the muscle cells of the coronary arteries. The clinical picture of this entity is a patent or locally occluded or stenosed coronary blood vessel, which is noncompliant. The short- and long-term patency of a graft on these rigid vessels is doubtful.

Assessment of graft patency following coronary artery bypass surgery

Several studies have investigated whether graft closure can be predicted with good results by post-operatively performing thallium scintigraphy. Greenberg *et al.* reported that, of 10 patients who had a positive stress scintigram, 8 (80%) had restenosis of one or more grafts, while the other two patients had > 75% stenosis in a native coronary artery [37]. In addition, 10 of 13 patients (77%) with a negative scintigram during optimal stress had complete revascularization on the post-operative coronary angiogram. This means an overall accuracy of 85%, which is similar to the accuracy of detecting coronary artery disease in patients without previous coronary surgery. Other studies reported similar values of thallium scintigraphy for the detection of graft patency (Table 9.3) [35,39,68–79].

Clinical implications

Thallium scintigraphy and PET imaging currently play an important role in the diagnosis of myocardial ischemia. However, the decision whether or not to revascularize is still mainly based on the presence of critical stenosis (> 70%) in the coronary arteries, as visualized on the coronary angiogram. Risk factors such as poor left ventricular function, age and other illnesses are also taken into account when a decision on coronary surgery has to be made. The previous review emphasizes that, with the differentiation between viable and nonviable myocardium, the potential for functional recovery of the myocardium after revascularization can be predicted quite accurately. This would mean that, in patients with a high risk of peri-operative mortality or morbidity, a good prediction can be made whether or not they will benefit from coronary surgery

Table 9.3. Thallium scintigraphy to predict the extent of myocardial revascularization

Study	Year	Technique	Pts	Patent graft/ no perfusion defect	Occluded graft/ perfusion defect	No perfusion defect/patent graft	Perfusion defect/ occluded graft
Ritchie [35]	1977	Tl-201 S-RD/R	20	26/30 (87%)	6/13 (46%)		
Greenberg [37]	1978	Tl-201 S-RD	25	10/13 (77%)[a]	8/10 (80%)[a]		
Sbarbaro [68]	1979	Tl-201 R+S-RD	15	10/11 (91%)[a]	3/4 (75%)[a]		
Wainwright [69]	1980	Tl-201 S-RD	48			61/77 (79%)	21/42 (50%)
Hirzel [39]	1980	Tl-201 S-RD	54	29/36 (81%)	32/47 (68%)		
Kolibash [70]	1980	Tl-201 S-RD	38	51/62 (82%)	15/34 (41%)		
Lösse [71]	1981	Tl-201 S-RD	60	72/79 (91%)	25/57 (44%)	72/104 (69%)	25/32 (78%)
Pfisterer [72]	1982	Tl-201 S-RD	55	30/33 (91%)[a]	12/16 (75%)[a]		11/18 (61%)
Usdin [73]	1983	Tl-201 S-RD	36			18/27 (67%)	5/9 (56%)
Engelstad [74]	1983	Tl-201 S-RD	24	40/48 (83%)	10/14 (71%)		
Rasmussen [75]	1984	Tl-201 S-RD	49	61/67 (91%)	15/19 (79%)	61/65 (94%)	(15/21 (71%)
Huikuri [76]	1987	Tl-201 S-RD	51	14/19 (74%)[a]	27/32 (84%)[a]	14/19 (74%)	27/32 (84%)
Zimmerman [77]	1988	Tl-201 S-RD	34			50/57 (88%)	9/11 (82%)
Naruse [78]	1988	Tl-201 R-RD	31[b]	30/32 (94%)	5/13 (39%)		
Kureshi [79]	1989	Tl-201 S-RD	17	NP	6/6 (100%)[a]		

[a] = patients; NP = not provided; R = rest; RD = redistribution; S = stress; [b] = 18 CABG, 13 PTCA.

in terms of long-term survival. As stated earlier, patients with poor left ventricular function and three-vessel disease may especially benefit from coronary surgery, compared to medical therapy. For practical purposes the following strategy could be used. In patients with an overall LVEF of more than 30% no further pre-operative evaluation is done, since the peri-operative mortality and morbidity are acceptable and neither thallium scintigraphy nor PET will change the indication for bypass surgery. In patients with severely impaired left ventricular function (LVEF <30%), the presence of viable myocardium is important to predict, to some extent, the outcome of the operation, both in short- and long-term survival. Patients with chronically depressed hibernating myocardium should not be denied an operation on the basis of poor ventricular function alone. The initial study with thallium-201, preferably with reinjection, may provide evidence of myocardial viability. If not, PET imaging may be indicated. Careful pre-operative evaluation is mandatory because of the peri-operative complications resulting in a prolonged stay in the intensive care. In view of the current reduction of health care budgets, this should be prevented if possible.

At this moment, both techniques for differentiation of viable and nonviable are equal with respect to sensitivity and specificity. This is also the case for the predictive value of both techniques for the outcome of coronary bypass surgery. However, the unavailability of PET is still an important drawback as are the high costs, compared to thallium scintigraphy. Moreover, the number of patients studied with PET is small.

Thallium scintigraphy can be useful in the post-operative follow-up of patients. The accuracy for detection of graft closure is similar to the accuracy of detection of coronary stenosis in patients without CABG.

Conclusion

The assessment of myocardial viability by either thallium-201 scintigraphy or FDG PET may be useful for the prediction of functional recovery and therefore for improvement in long-term survival rates and the decrement in the number of events following coronary artery bypass surgery. It may be especially useful in identifying patients in high risk groups, such as patients with impaired left ventricular function, who may benefit the most from coronary revascularization. Proper evaluation of patients with poor left ventricular function will allow operations on patients who otherwise would have been rejected on the basis of poor left ventricular function alone. It may also select out patients in whom no improvement of ventricular function is to be expected. However, caution should remain, since despite the number of published studies concerning this topic, no large prospective multicentre trials have yet been performed.

References

1. Favaloro RG. Saphenous vein autograft replacement of severe segmental coronary occlusion: Operative technique. Ann Thorac Surg 1968; 5: 334–9.
2. Myers WO, Schaff HV, Gersh BJ, Fisher KD, Kosinski AS, Mock MD *et al.* Improved survival of surgically treated patients with triple vessel coronary artery disease and severe angina pectoris. A report from the Coronary Artery Surgery Study (CASS) registry. J Thorac Cardiovasc Surg 1989; 97: 487–95.
3. American College of Cardiology/American Heart Association. ACC/AHA guidelines and indications for coronary artery bypass graft surgery. A report of the ACC/AHA Task Force on Assessment of Diagnostic and Therapeutic Cardiovascular Procedures (Subcommittee on Coronary Artery Bypass Graft Surgery). Circulation 1991; 83: 1125–73.
4. Horn HR, Teichholz LE, Cohn PF, Herman MV, Gorlin R. Augmentation of left ventricular contraction in coronary artery disease by an inotropic catecholamine. The epinephrine ventriculogram. Circulation 1974; 49: 1063–71.
5. Rozanski A, Berman D, Gray R, Diamond G, Raymond M, Pranse J *et al.* Preoperative prediction of reversible myocardial asynergy by postexercise radionuclide ventriculography. N Engl J Med 1982; 307: 212–6.
6. Braunwald E, Rutherford JD. Reversible ischemic left ventricular dysfunction: Evidence for the 'hibernating myocardium'. J Am Coll Cardiol 1986; 8: 1467–70.
7. Rahimtoola SH. The hibernating myocardium. Am Heart J 1989; 117: 211–21.
8. Dilsizian V, Bonow RO, Cannon RO 3d, Tracey CM, Vitale DF, McIntosh CL *et al.* The effect of coronary artery bypass grafting on left ventricular systolic function at rest: Evidence for preoperative subclinical myocardial ischemia. Am J Cardiol 1988; 61: 1248–54.
9. Elefteriades JA, Tolis G Jr, Levi E, Mills LK, Zaret BL. Coronary artery bypass grafting in severe left ventricular dysfunction: Excellent survival with improved ejection fraction and functional state. J Am Coll Cardiol 1993; 22: 1411–7.
10. Elami A, Uretzky G, Appelbaum A, Gotsman MS, Borman JB. Improved functional results following myocardial revascularization in patients with left ventricular dysfunction. J Cardiovasc Surg (Torino) 1987; 28: 61–7.
11. Brunken R, Tillisch J, Schwaiger M, Child JS, Marshall R, Mandelkern M *et al.* Regional perfusion, glucose metabolism, and wall motion in patients with chronic electrocardiographic Q-wave infarctions: Evidence for persistence of viable tissue in some infarct regions by positron emission tomography. Circulation 1986; 73: 951–63.
12. Marwick TH, MacIntyre WJ, Lafont A, Nemec JJ, Salcedo EE. Metabolic responses of hibernating and infarcted myocardium to revascularisation. A follow-up study of regional perfusion, function, and metabolism. Circulation 1992; 85: 1347–53.
13. Bourassa MG, Lesperance J, Campeau L, Saltiel J. Fate of left ventricular contraction following aortocoronary venous grafts. Early and late postoperative modifications. Circulation 1972; 46: 724–30.
14. Proudfit WL, Bruschke AV, Sones FM Jr. Natural history of obstructive coronary artery disease: Ten-year study of 601 nonsurgical cases. Prog Cardiovasc Dis 1978; 21: 53–78.
15. Kalmar P, Irrgang E. Cardiac surgery in Germany during 1991. A report by the German Society for Thoracic and Cardiovascular Surgery. Thorac Cardiovasc Surg 1992; 40: 163–5.
16. Christakis GT, Weisel RD, Fremes SE, Ivanov J, David TE, Goldman BS *et al.* Coronary artery bypass grafting in patients with poor ventricular function. Cardiovascular Surgeons of the University of Toronto. J Thorac Cardiovasc Surg 1992; 103: 1083–91; discussion 1091–2.
17. Bounous EP, Mark DB, Pollock BG, Hlatky MA, Harrel FE Jr, Lee KL *et al.* Surgical survival benefits for coronary disease patients with left ventricular dysfunction. Circulation 1988; 78: I151–7.
18. Coronary artery surgery study (CASS): a randomized trial of coronary artery bypass surgery. Survival data. Circulation 1983; 68: 939–50.
19. Califf RM, Harrell FE Jr, Lee KL, Rankin JS, Mark DB, Hlatky MA *et al.* Changing efficacy of coronary revascularization. Implications for patient selection. Circulation 1988; 78: I185–91.

20. Veterans Affairs Coronary Artery Bypass Surgery Cooperative Study Group. Eighteen-year follow up in the Veterans Affairs Cooperative Study of Coronary Artery Bypass Surgery for stable angina. Circulation 1992; 86: 121–30.
21. Bell MR, Gersh BJ, Schaff HV, Holmes DR Jr, Fisher LD, Alderman DL et al. Effect of completeness of revascularization on long-term outcome of patients with three-vessel disease undergoing coronary artery bypass surgery. A report from the Coronary Artery Surgery Study (CASS) Registry. Circulation 1992; 86: 446–57.
22. Loop FD, Lytle BW, Cosgrove DM, Stewart RW, Goormastic M, Williams GW et al. Influence of the internal-mammary-artery graft on 10-year survival and other cardiac events. N Engl J Med 1986; 314: 1–6.
23. Jones EL, Weinraub WS, Craver JM, Guyton RA, Cohen CL. Coronary bypass surgery: Is the operation different today? J Thorac Cardiovasc Surg 1991; 101: 108–15.
24. Maddahi J, Garcia EV, Berman DS, Waxman A, Swan HJ, Forrester J. Improved noninvasive assessment of coronary artery disease by quantitative analysis of regional stress myocardial distribution and washout of thallium-201. Circulation 1981; 64: 924–35.
25. Tamaki N, Yonekura Y, Mukai T, Kodama S, Kadota K, Kambara H et al. Stress thallium-201 transaxial emission computed tomography: Quantitative versus qualitative analysis for evaluation of coronary artery disease. J Am Coll Cardiol 1984; 4: 1213–21.
26. Pohost GM, Zir LM, Moore RH, McKusick KA, Guiney TE, Beller GA. Differentiation of transiently ischemic from infarcted myocardium by serial imaging after a single dose of thallium-201. Circulation 1977; 55: 294–302.
27. Dilsizian V, Bacharach SL, Perrone-Filardi P, Arrighi JM, Maurea S, Bonow RO. Concordance and disconcordance between rest-redistribution thallium imaging and thallium reinjection after stress-redistribution imaging for assessing viable myocardium: Comparison with metabolic activity by PET [abstract]. Circulation 1991; 84 (4 suppl II): II89.
28. Dondi M, Tartagni F, Fallani F, Fanti S, Marengo M, DiTomasso I et al. A comparison of rest sestamibi and rest-redistribution thallium single photon emission tomography: Possible implications for myocardial viability detection in infarcted patients. Eur J Nucl Med 1993; 20: 26–31.
29. Gutman J, Berman DS, Freeman M, Rozanski A, Maddahi J, Waxman A et al. Time to completed redistribution of thallium-201 in exercise myocardial scintigraphy: Relationship to the degree of coronary artery stenosis. Am Heart J 1983; 106: 989–95.
30. Cloninger KG, DePuey EG, Garcia EV, Roubin GS, Robbins WL, Nody A et al. Incomplete redistribution in delayed thallium-201 single photon emission computed tomographic (SPECT) images: An overestimation of myocardial scarring. J Am Coll Cardiol 1988; 12: 955–63.
31. Kiat H, Berman DS, Maddahi J, De Yang L, Van Train K, Rozanski A et al. Late reversibility of tomographic myocardial thallium-201 defects: An accurate marker of myocardial viability. J Am Coll Cardiol 1988; 12: 1456–63.
32. Dilsizian V, Rocco TP, Freedman NM, Leon MB, Bonow RO. Enhanced detection of ischemic but viable myocardium by the reinjection of thallium after stress-redistribution imaging. N Engl J Med 1990; 323: 141–6.
33. Van Eck-Smit BLF, van der Wall EE, Kuijper AFM, Zwinderman AH, Pauwels EK. Immediate thallium-201 reinjection following stress imaging: A time-saving approach for detection of myocardial viability. J Nucl Med 1993; 34: 737–43.
34. Rozanski A, Berman DS, Gray R, Levy R, Raymond M, Maddahi J et al. Use of thallium-201 redistribution scintigraphy in the preoperative differentiation of reversible and nonreversible myocardial asynergy. Circulation 1981; 64: 936–44.
35. Ritchie JL, Narahara KA, Trobaugh GB, Williams DL, Hamilton GW. Thallium-201 myocardial imaging before and after coronary revascularization: Assessment of regional myocardial blood flow and graft patency. Circulation 1977; 56: 830–6.
36. Verani MS, Marcus ML, Spoto G, Rossi NP, Ehrhardt JC, Razzak MA. Thallium-201 myocardial perfusion scintigrams in the evaluation of aorto-coronary saphenous bypass surgery. J Nucl Med 1978; 19: 765–72.
37. Greenberg BH, Hart R, Botvinick EH, Werner JA, Brundage BH, Shames DM et al. Thallium-

201 myocardial perfusion scintigraphy to evaluate patients after coronary bypass surgery. Am J Cardiol 1978; 42: 167–76.

38. Robinson PS, Williams BT, Webb-Peploe MM, Crowther A, Coltart DJ. Thallium-201 myocardial imaging in assessment of results of aortocoronary bypass surgery. Br Heart J 1979; 42: 455–62.

39. Hirzel HO, Nuesch K, Sialer G, Horst W, Krayenbuhl HP. Thallium-201 exercise myocardial imaging to evaluate myocardial perfusion after coronary bypass surgery. Br Heart J 1980; 43: 426–35.

40. Gibson RS, Watson DD, Taylor GJ, Crosby IK, Wellons HL, Holt ND *et al.* Prospective assessment of regional myocardial perfusion before and after coronary revascularization surgery by quantitative thallium-201 scintigraphy. J Am Coll Cardiol 1983; 1: 804–15.

41. Brundage BH, Massie BM, Botvinick EH. Improved regional ventricular function after successful surgical revascularization. J Am Coll Cardiol 1984; 3: 902–8.

42. Liu P, Kiess MC, Okada RD, Block PC, Strauss HW, Pohost GM *et al.* The persistent defect on exercise thallium imaging and its fate after myocardial revascularization: Does it represent scar or ischemia? Am Heart J 1985; 110: 996–1001.

43. Tamaki N, Yonekura Y, Yamashita K, Senda M, Saji H, Konishi Y *et al.* Value of rest-stress myocardial positron tomography using nitrogen-13 ammonia for the preoperative prediction of reversible asynergy. J Nucl Med 1989; 30: 1302–10.

44. Ohtani H, Tamaki N, Yonekura Y, Mohiuddin IH, Hirata K, Ban T *et al.* Value of thallium-201 reinjection after delayed SPECT imaging for predicting reversible ischemia after coronary artery bypass grafting. Am J Cardiol 1990; 66: 394–9.

45. Ohtani H, Tamaki N, Mohiuddin IH, Yonekura Y, Konishi J, Hirata K *et al.* Minimal redistribution of thallium-201 representing reversible ischemia after coronary bypass surgery: Value of quantitative analysis of exercise thallium-201 SPECT [Japanese]. J Cardiol 1991; 21: 835–46.

46. Tamaki N, Ohtani H, Yamashita K, Magata Y, Yonekura Y, Nohara R *et al.* Metabolic activity in the areas of new-fill-in after thallium-201 reinjection: Comparison with positron emission tomography using fluorine-18-deoxyglucose. J Nucl Med 1991; 32: 673–8.

47. Contini GA, Calbiani B, Antonelli AM, Campodonico R, Astorri E, Fesani F. Exercise thallium-201 myocardial scintigraphy before and after coronary artery bypass surgery. In press.

48. Berger BC, Watson DD, Burwell LR, Crosby IK, Wellons HA, Teates CD *et al.* Redistribution of thallium at rest in patients with stable and unstable angina and the effect of coronary artery bypass surgery. Circulation 1979; 60: 1114–25.

49. Iskandrian AS, Hakki AH, Kane SA, Goel IP, Mundth ED, Segal BL. Rest and redistibution thallium-201 myocardial scintigraphy to predict improvement in left ventricular function after coronary arterial bypass grafting. Am J Cardiol 1983; 51: 1312–6.

50. Mori T, Minamiji K, Kurogane H, Ogawa K, Yoshida Y. Rest-injected thallium-201 imaging for assessing viability of severe asynergic regions. J Nucl Med 1991; 32: 1718–24.

51. Naruse H, Ohyanagi M, Iwasaki T, Miyamoto T, Fukuchi M. Preoperative evaluation of myocardial viability by thallium-201 imaging in patients with old myocardial infarction who underwent coronary revascularization. Ann Nucl Med 1992; 6: 51–8.

52. Giubbini R, Milan E, Rossini PL, Alfieri O, Ferrari R, Metra M *et al.* Combined evaluation of perfusion and function for the identification of viable myocardium. J Nucl Biol Med 1992; 36 (2 Suppl): 126–9.

53. Ragosta M, Beller GA, Watson DD, Kaul S, Gimple LW. Quantitative planar rest-redistribution ^{201}Tl imaging in detection of myocardial viability and prediction of improvement in left ventricular function after coronary artery bypass surgery in patients with severely depressed left ventricular function. Circulation 1993; 87: 1630–41.

54. Coleman PS, Metherall JA, Pandian NG, Shea NL, Oates E, Konstam MA *et al.* Predicting enhanced regional ventricular function post-revascularization: Comparison of thallium-201 and Sestamibi in patients with left ventricular dysfunction [abstract]. Circulation 1992; 86 (4 Suppl I): I108.

55. Kuijper AF, Niemeyer MG, D'haene EG, van der Wall EE, Pauwels EK. Stress-reinjection

thallium-201 scintigraphy: Prediction of effect of coronary artery bypass grafting on regional myocardial perfusion [abstract]. J Am Coll Cardiol 1993; 21 (Suppl A): 389A.

56. Zimmerman R, Tillmanns H, Rauch B, Mall G, Hagl S. Structural alterations and the effect of coronary revascularization in myocardial regions with mild-to-moderate or severe persistent thallium-201 defects [abstract]. Circulation 1993; 88 (4 Suppl I): I199.

57. Tillisch J, Brunken R, Marshall R, Schwaiger M, Mandelkern M, Phelps M *et al.* Reversibility of cardiac wall-motion abnormalities predicted by positron tomography. N Engl J Med 1986; 314: 884–8.

58. Tamaki N, Yonekura Y, Yamashita K, Saji H, Magata Y, Senda M *et al.* Positron emission tomography using fluorine-18 deoxyglucose in evaluation of coronary artery bypass grafting. Am J Cardiol 1989; 64: 860–5.

59. Lucignani G, Paolini G, Landoni C, Zuccari M, Paganelli G, Galli L *et al.* Presurgical identification of hibernating myocardium by combined use of technetium-99m hexakis 2-methoxyisobutylisonitrile single photon emission tomography and fluorine-18 fluoro-2-deoxy-D-glucose positron emission tomography in patients with coronary artery disease. Eur J Nucl Med 1992; 19: 874–81.

60. Schelbert HR, Schwaiger M. Positron emission tomography in human myocardial ischemia. Herz 1987; 12: 22–40.

61. Al-Aouar ZR, Eitzman D, Hepner A, Lee KS, Kirsh MM, Hicks RJ *et al.* PET assessment of myocardial tissue viability: University of Michigan experience [abstract]. J Nucl Med 1990; 31 (5 Suppl): 801.

62. Tamaki N, Yonekura Y, Yamashita K, Ohtani H, Hirata K, Ban T *et al.* Prediction of reversible ischemia after coronary artery bypass grafting by positron emission tomography. J Cardiol 1991; 21: 193–201.

63. Marwick TH, Nemec JJ, Lafont A, Salcedo EE, MacIntyre WJ. Prediction of postexercise fluor-18 deoxyglucose positron emission tomography of improvement in exercise capacity after revascularization. Am J Cardiol 1992; 69: 854–9.

64. Tamaki N. Assessment of myocardial viability by use of multiple clinical parameters and effect on prognosis. Coronary Artery Dis 1993; 4: 521–8.

65. Gropler RJ, Geltman EM, Sampathkumaran K, Perez JE, Schechtman KB, Conversano A *et al.* Comparison of carbon-11-acetate with fluorine-18-fluorodeoxyglucose for delineating viable myocardium by positron emission tomography. J Am Coll Cardiol 1993; 22: 1587–97.

66. Eitzman D, Al-Aouar Z, Kanter H, Vom Dahl J, Kirsh M, Deet GM *et al.* Clinical outcome of patients with advanced coronary artery disease after viability studies with positron emission tomography. J Am Coll Cardiol 1992; 20: 559–65.

67. Breisblatt WM, Stein KL, Wolfe CJ, Follansbee WP, Capozzi J, Armitage JM *et al.* Acute myocardial dysfunction and recovery: A common occurrence after coronary bypass surgery. J Am Coll Cardiol 1990; 15: 1261–9.

68. Sbarbaro JA, Karunaratne H, Cantez S, Harper PV, Resnekov L. Thallium-201 imaging in assessment of aortocoronary bypass graft patency. Br Heart J 1979; 42: 553–61.

69. Wainwright RJ, Brennand-Roper DA, Maisey MN, Sowton E. Exercise thallium-201 myocardial scintigraphy in the follow-up of aortocoronary bypass graft surgery. Br Heart J 1980; 43: 56–66.

70. Kolibash AJ, Call TD, Bush CA, Tetalman MR, Lewis RP. Myocardial perfusion as an indicator of graft patency after coronary artery bypass surgery. Circulation 1980; 61: 882–7.

71. Lösse B, Von Lierde C, Rafflenbeul D, Kronert H, Bircks W, Feinendegen LE *et al.* Wert der Thallium-201-Myocardszintigraphie für die Beurteilung des Funktionszustandes aorto-koronarer Bypass-Gefäße. Z Kardiol 1981; 70: 231–7.

72. Pfisterer M, Emmenegger H, Schmitt HE, Muller-Brand J, Hasse J, Gradel E *et al.* Accuracy of serial myocardial perfusion scintigraphy with thallium-201 for prediction of graft patency early and late after coronary artery bypass surgery. A controlled prospective study. Circulation 1982; 66: 1017–24.

73. Usdin JP, Vasile N, Cinotti L, Meignan M, Legendre T, Larde P *et al.* Evaluation atraumatique

de la permeabilitè des pontages aorto-coronariens par la tomodensitometrie et la scintigraphie myocardique à l'effort. Arch Mal Coeur Vaiss 1983; 76: 183–92.

74. Engelstad BL, Wagner S, Herfkens R, Botvinick E, Brundage B, Lipton M. Evaluation of the post-coronary artery bypass patient by myocardial perfusion scintigraphy and computed tomography. AJR Am J Roentgenol 1983; 141: 507–12.

75. Rasmussen SL, Nielsen SL, Amtorp O, Folke K, Fritz-Hansen P. 201-Thallium imaging as an indicator of graft patency after coronary artery bypass surgery. Eur Heart J 1984; 5: 494–9.

76. Huikuri HV, Ikaheimo MJ, Korhonen UR, Heikkila J, Takkunen JT. Thallium scintigraphy in prediction of occlusion of bypass grafts in asymptomatic and symptomatic patients. Acta Med Scand 1987; 222: 311–8.

77. Zimmermann R, Tillmanns H, Knapp WH, Neumann FJ, Saggau W, Kübler W. Noninvasive assessment of coronary artery bypass patency: Determination of myocardial thallium-201 washout rates. Eur Heart J 1988; 9: 319–27.

78. Naruse H, Kawamoto H, Ohyanagi M, Hazzaki R, Yasutomi N, Iwasaki T *et al.* Indications for coronary revascularization and the postoperative evaluations using Tl-201 exercise myocardial scintigraphy and a bull's eye display [Japanese]. J Cardiol 1988; 18: 79–88.

79. Kureshi SA, Tamaki N, Yonekura Y, Koide H, Konishi Y, Ban T *et al.* Value of stress thallium-201 emission tomography for predicting improvement after coronary bypass grafting and assessing graft patency. Jpn Heart J 1989; 30: 287–99.

10. When is myocardial viability a clinically relevant issue?

Summary and perspectives

ABDULMASSIH S. ISKANDRIAN & ERNST E. VAN DER WALL

Left ventricular (LV) dysfunction may be reversible or irreversible after coronary revascularization [1–5]. If the dysfunction is due to stunning or hibernation, recovery is observed, but if it is due to scarring, no recovery occurs [5–7]. Stunning differs from hibernation in that recovery can occur in stunning with no revascularization since, by definition, it represents a dysfunction following an episode of ischemia, despite normalization of myocardial blood flow [6]. On the other hand, dysfunction related to hibernation is a chronic process due to chronic reduction in the resting myocardial blood flow. Unlike stunning, there are no animal models to study chronic hibernation and there are no serial studies in patients with hibernation to determine the chronicity of the disorder or whether 'severity' of the hibernation is stable over time [8]. It is quite conceivable that, even in patients with hibernation, there are episodes of superimposed stunning due to baseline changes in coronary blood flow or stress-induced myocardial ischemia, secondary to increase in myocardial oxygen demand. Pure stunning is unusual and may be seen in patients with severe coronary artery disease (CAD) after strenuous exercise, in patients with unstable angina pectoris or patients undergoing percutaneous transluminal coronary angioplasty. Hibernation can be viewed as a process of a flow-contraction match due to down-regulation of contractile function in order to reduce energy expenditure and preserve myocyte survival. The dysfunction is an adaptive process to decrease myocardial oxygen demand [6–8].

Apart from stunning and hibernation, a myocardial segment may have contractile dysfunction due to myocardial scar; if the infarction is nontransmural, that segment of the myocardium may have a combination of normal and scar tissue. Therefore, in any given patient and any given segment, a combination of normal, scar, hibernation and stunned myocardium may coexist in different proportions.

There are three issues that need to be addressed in patients with LV dysfunction: First, who are the patients who need viability assessment? Second, what is the optimum method to detect viability? Third, what are the factors that govern the recovery of LV function after coronary revascularization?

A.S. Iskandrian and E.E. van der Wall (eds): Myocardial viability, 179–192.
© 1994 *Kluwer Academic Publishers.*

Patient selection for viability studies

There are two groups of patients in whom viability studies are indicated: those with severe global LV dysfunction due to CAD and, more importantly, those patients with regional dysfunction after acute myocardial infarction. It is needless to mention that viability should not be looked for in patients with normal or near normal LV function.

Patients with severe LV dysfunction, especially those with an ejection fraction (EF) of <30%, may be symptomatic or asymptomatic. The symptoms may be those of congestive heart failure or angina pectoris. If angina pectoris is moderate or severe and is interfering with the lifestyle of the patient, coronary revascularization may be indicated without the need of viability studies. In heart failure centers, roughly 50% of patients have LV dysfunction due to CAD and the remaining patients, LV dysfunction due to primary cardiomyopathy or valvular heart disease. Obviously, it is in the subgroup of patients with LV dysfunction due to CAD (ischemic cardiomyopathy) that viability studies are indicated. It is probably true that most patients, including those with LV dysfunction, can survive coronary artery bypass surgery (CABG), although the surgical risk is higher in these patients than in those with normal LV function. The important question to be asked is whether these patients will improve symptomatically and whether their prognosis will be better after coronary revascularization. If patients with *reversible* LV dysfunction are appropriately identified, their functional status and prognosis are significantly better after coronary revascularization than with medical therapy. On the other hand, in patients with *irreversible* LV dysfunction due to myocardial scarring, the functional class and prognosis are similar with medical therapy and surgical revascularization.

The second group of patients are those with a fairly large area of myocardial dysfunction after myocardial infarction. The issue is often more pertinent in patients after thrombolytic therapy, who have residual flow-limiting stenosis [2]. The work by Sabia *et al.*, injecting microbubbles directly into the coronary arteries at the time of catheterization to study coronary microcirculation, suggested that collaterals may preserve viability for some time after acute infarction and that functional improvement is observed after successful angioplasty [9]. Since the dysfunction is regional in these patients, coronary angioplasty rather than surgery is the procedure most often recommended. However, similar to the patients requiring surgery, the indication is that angioplasty will improve the contractile function of the infarcted segment rather than improving the symptoms. Needless to say, angioplasty is indicated in patients with recurrent ischemia, evidenced as recurrent angina or by stress testing. The number of patients with recent myocardial infarction, potentially requiring early revascularization because of residual viable myocardium, is likely to increase due to a decline in early mortality and increased use of early thrombolytic therapy. As the cost of early diagnosis and care are likely to increase, cost-effective techniques to identify appropriate candidates are important. In summary, the indications for coronary revascularization in patients with LV dysfunction are two-fold; to alleviate symptoms and improve prognosis. This holds true both for patients with global and those with regional dysfunction, regardless of the severity of symptoms.

In the experience of many investigators in this field, viability studies are necessary in approximately 5–10% of patients who are referred to busy nuclear cardiology laboratories for work-up. The percentage may be higher in patients after acute infarction, especially after thrombolytic therapy and in specialized centers dealing with patients with congestive heart failure [4].

Which technique should be used to assess viability?

Diagnostic techniques that predict improvement in LV function should have high positive as well as negative predictive values. For example, a diagnostic technique that identifies scar but not viable myocardium will have a high negative predictive value but a low positive predictive value. This is not unlike a diagnostic technique that is good for excluding CAD but is poor in predicting the presence of CAD. This issue is also important in patient selection. For example, if patients with predominantly irreversible LV dysfunction are included, the positive predictive value of the test may not be precisely known, although the test may be correct in most cases in predicting those with irreversible LV dysfunction!

The available methods for assessing myocardial viability include demonstration of *functional* integrity by echocardiography, magnetic resonance imaging, and contrast angiography or demonstration of *metabolic* integrity by scintigraphic techniques [10–27].

1. Functional assessment
   - Echocardiography
   - Magnetic resonance imaging
   - Contrast angiography
2. Metabolic assessment
   - Myocardial scintigraphy
     - Single photon emission tomography
     - Positron emission tomography

The choice between these methods may depend on the expertise and availability of resources, especially those of expensive technologies such as positron emission tomography and magnetic resonance imaging. Therefore, what may work best in one center may be different in another. Interventional techniques in the cardiac catheterization laboratory, using post-extrasystolic accentuation and nitroglycerin intervention left ventriculography have not been widely used or accepted, possibly because of the invasive nature of these interventions. Nevertheless, coronary angiography has a central role in patient management because the decision regarding coronary revascularization relies heavily on the suitability of the coronary arteries for corrective surgery or angioplasty. Coronary angiography is also useful in the assessment of collateral vessels; however, there is discordance between the angiographic appearance of collaterals and their function, as discussed by Kaul in the chapter of echocardiography. Most collaterals are 50–100 μ in dimension and may not be angiographically visible. Of most concern is that even well-developed collaterals by angiography may not predict the status of myocardial viability.

Several methods have been used with positron emission tomography, such as studying the washout of rubidium-82 and the assessment of the water content of the myocardium, but the method most widely used and tested is based on assessment of metabolism and flow using two different tracers; fluorine-18 (F-18) labeled with deoxyglucose (FDG) and nitrogen-13 (N-13) labeled with ammonia are the two commonly used tracers [6,13,18,19]. The usefulness of FDG in diabetic patients and early after acute myocardial infarction is not clearly established. A more recent and novel method discussed by Bergmann relies on the study of myocardial oxidative metabolism using C-11 acetate. Based on receiver operating characteristic curve analysis, the results by acetate analysis were more robust than those based on the flow or FDG (or both) in predicting the recovery of contractile function. The concept is based on the principle that oxidative metabolism is maintained in viable myocardium and its loss indicates myocardial necrosis. Although there is a parallel relationship between oxidative metabolism and myocardial flow, this relationship is not strong enough, probably because of changes in oxygen extraction. Normal function and viability are present when the myocardial blood flow is over 80% of the normal value at rest. Disparity between flow and viability may occur when the flow is reduced between 30% and 80% of the baseline normal value. Evidence of viability is certainly unlikely when the flow is reduced to below 30% of the baseline normal value.

Scintigraphic techniques rely heavily on the principle that integrity of the cell membrane is the hallmark of viable myocardium [10,21]. The use of thallium and, more recently, technetium-labeled imaging agents are the prototypes. One such method is rest-redistribution imaging [20,22]. With this approach, the following patterns were found to be predictive of functional recovery: 1) normal initial uptake, 2) reversible defect, and 3) mild fixed defect. While it is easy to understand why reversible defects show improvement in contractile function (as these segments represent hibernation), it is not clear why 'normal' segments or mild fixed defects show similar improvement. Whether these segments represent stunned myocardium or whether some redistribution is present but cannot be detected is unclear. It is also possible that the normal segments are only relatively normal. Parenthetically, mild fixed thallium defects often have a matched reduction of flow and metabolism by positron emission tomography. Because of the advantage of concomitant information on reversible ischemia and viability, protocols that combine stress with rest imaging are most often used for detecting overall viability. In this respect, several protocols have been proposed, such as the stress-4-hour redistribution-reinjection protocol [23–25], and the stress-immediate reinjection approach [24]. Dilsizian *et al.* [23] showed that the thallium stress-4-hour redistribution-reinjection protocol yielded the most comprehensive information on myocardial viability, similar to the information obtained by positron emission tomography. Van Eck-Smit *et al.* [24] clearly demonstrated that reinjection of thallium-201 immediately post-stress imaging, followed by imaging 1 hour later, proved a time-saving and patient-convenient approach to assess viability.

It is possible that modification of imaging protocols with technetium-99m Sestamibi may provide comparable results. These modifications include the use of nitroglycerin before imaging, acquisition of gated images (analysis of diastolic and systolic images), assessment of wall thickening, quantitative assessment of the tracer uptake, simultaneous assessment of function by first-pass radionuclide angiography delaying image acquisition to longer-than-usual times (i.e. 2–3 hours rather than 30–60 minutes) after injection or the use of rest-redistribution festamibi imaging similar to rest-redistribution thallium-201 imaging. More work is needed in this area but, for now, thallium-201 is preferable over Sestamibi. Other technetium-99m labeled imaging agents such as tetrofosmin and furifosmin (Q-12) have not yet been studied for viability assessment, however, experience indicates that technetium-99m teboroxime is not suitable for viability assessment. The use of I-123 IPPA (iodophenylpentadecanoic acid) is now undergoing Phase III clinical trials in the U.S. to assess myocardial viability [14]. The metabolism of this long chain fatty acid is different in normal myocardium than in ischemic myocardium. The clearance is bi-exponential: most of the clearance is early due to β-oxidation and the slow clearance is due to incorporation into triglyceride and phospholipid pools. The clearance in ischemic myocardium is slow, due to predominant incorporation of the fatty acid into the phospholipid and triglyceride pools. This pattern of differential 'washout' may, therefore, be used by serial imaging to determine the presence of hibernating myocardium.

At the Philadelphia Heart Institute, the ability of dynamic SPECT I-123 IPPA imaging was examined to detect myocardial viability in 18 patients with LV dysfunction. Serial 180° SPECT images (5 sets, 8 minutes each) were obtained starting at 4 minutes after injection of 2–6 mCi of IPPA at rest [14]. The uptake in each of 20 segments per patient was compared to that of rest-redistribution thallium-201 images. The rest-redistribution and the IPPA images were abnormal in all patients. In 10 patients the thallium images showed evidence of fixed defects and, in 8 patients, both reversible and fixed defects. On the other hand, with IPPA imaging, 2 patients showed fixed defects, and 16 patients had reversible defects or both fixed and reversible defect. Of the 360 segments studied by thallium imaging, 189 were normal, 36 were reversible, and 135 were fixed (47 mild and 88 severe). With IPPA images there were 169 normal segments, 118 reversible and 73 fixed. More reversible defects were detected by IPPA than by thallium imaging. Of the 69 segments with reversible IPPA but fixed thallium defects, the defects were mild in 47 segments (> 50% uptake of normal) and severe in 22 segments. In 12 patients the EF was repeated after coronary

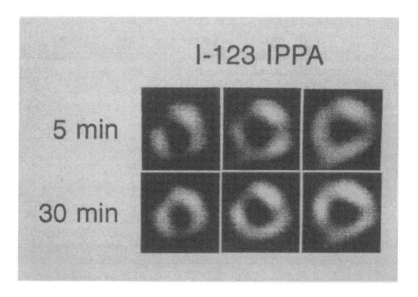

Figure 10.1. Serial I-123 IPPA images in a patient with left ventricular dysfunction. Short axis slices are shown. There are multiple reversible defects. This patient had improvement of ejection fraction after coronary artery bypass surgery.

revascularization and improved by $\geq$ 5% in 6 of 12 patients. The patients with improved EF had more reversible IPPA segments per patient than patients who did not show improvement (9 versus 4).

Thus, dynamic I-123 IPPA imaging is a promising new technique to assess myocardial viability. IPPA evidence of hibernation predicts improvement in EF after coronary revascularization. The slightly more reversible defects seen with IPPA than with rest-redistribution thallium imaging may indicate our inability to detect redistribution when defects are mild (and hence, the need for better quantitative methods), or it may indicate that some redistribution has already occurred by the time the first set of rest thallium-201 images were obtained – usually 20–30 minutes after injection. It is possible that these images should be obtained earlier, for example 5 minutes after injection. It should be mentioned parenthetically that the first set of IPPA images were obtained 4 minutes after rest injection. In general, the IPPA images were of better quality than the thallium images and most reversible defects were apparent by the third set of images (Figure 10.1). The entire protocol lasts less than 1 hour, which is faster than other comparable protocols.

The use of dobutamine echocardiography is another useful technique for the assessment of both myocardial thickening and wall motion. Because wall motion is load-dependent and is affected by tethering and translational movement due to respiration, assessment of thickening is probably more important. The presence of myocardial thickening denotes the presence of viable myocardium, however, a lack of thickening may still be compatible with viability. The dose of dobutamine may vary: a low dose may not be ideal for all patients. The dose may depend on the extent of necrosis and the presence or absence of a flow-limiting lesion in the infarct artery. In general, improvement or deterioration in wall motion or thickening may be markers of viability. Improvement is probably more common with stunned than hibernating myocardium.

In a broader context, the lack of infarct expansion or regional thinning may also be indirect markers of viable myocardium. Contrast echocardiography is a promising technique but, at the present time, requires intracoronary administration of micro air bubbles. These bubbles remain entirely within the intravascular space and reflect the status of the microvascular perfusion in that region. Clinical studies have shown that, in patients with acute myocardial infarction, the extent of the collateral bed supplied by collateral flow (depicted by contrast echocardiography) is a good predictor of functional recovery after coronary angioplasty. Importantly, no correlation is seen between angiographic appearance of collaterals and the spatial extent of collateral perfusion defined by contrast echocardiography. Early studies were done in patients with occluded infarct-related arteries with injection of microbubbles into the contralateral artery. More recent studies have shown similar conclusions in patients with open infarct arteries. Experimental studies, however, have shown that, in the absence of coronary vasodilation (such as dipyridamole), the region of 'no-flow' underestimates infarct size in the presence of a patent infarct artery. However, in the presence of a coronary vasodilator, the perfusion defect size corresponds to the infarct size, while the regions with contrast uptake depict viable myocardium.

Assessment of wall motion and thickening at baseline with dobutamine infusion can be obtained with even better resolution with magnetic resonance imaging. Good anatomical and temporal resolution, three-dimensional capabilities, unlimited field of view, and the possibility of *in vivo* measurement of myocardial biochemistry are unique features of magnetic resonance imaging. To date, the technique is only sparsely used for this purpose, possibly because of the long scanning time and relatively high cost of the equipment. Recent developments, like high-speed subsecond imaging, will have a significant impact on the time required for the study and will potentially reduce costs. Magnetic resonance imaging may prove valuable in the detection of a wide range of pathophysiological entities such as flow, perfusion, wall motion and cardiac metabolism.

Which technique should be used?

In institutions that have access to positron imaging tomography, this technique is probably the method of choice but, since it is unavailable in most medical centers, stress-reinjection or rest-redistribution thallium imaging are the most popular methods (Figure 10.2). The results of the rest-redistribution thallium study in 21 patients with severe LV dysfunction by Ragosta *et al.* are summarized in Tables 10.1–10.3 (22). Important findings from the study include

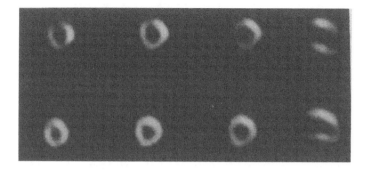

Figure 10.2. Rest-redistribution thallium images showing reversible defects. This patient had improvement of ejection fraction after coronary artery bypass surgery.

Table 10.1. Definitions of myocardial viability by rest-redistribution thallium-201

Type	Initial uptake	Redistribution
Normal	Normal	Normal
	Mild	Complete
	Severe	Complete
Mild decrease	Mild	Partial
	Severe	Partial
	Mild	No
Severe decrease	Severe	No

Adopted from Ragosta *et al.* [22].

Table 10.2. The relation between myocardial viability and improvement of asynergy after surgery (*n*: 176 segments)

	Preoperative viability	Improvement after surgery
Normal	(*n*: 58)	62%
Mild decrease	(*n*: 83)	54%
Severe decrease	(*n*: 35)	23%

Adopted from Ragosta *et al.* [22].

Table 10.3. The relation between preoperative wall motion and improvement after surgery.

	Preoperative	Improvement
Mild hypokinesia	(*n*: 74)	19%
Severe hypokinesia	(*n*: 82)	52%
Akinesia	(*n*: 87)	46%
Dyskinesia	(*n*: 7)	86%

Adopted from Ragosta *et al.* [22].

the presence of viable myocardium even in segments with severe wall motion abnormality and improvement in function after coronary revascularization even in segments with severe dysfunction.

What are the factors that affect the degree of improvement of LV function after coronary revascularization?

The factors that affect the degree of improvement of left ventricular function after coronary revascularization are:

1. The size extent of viable myocardium determined by pre-operative evaluation
2. The timing of post-revascularization assessment
3. The method of assessment
4. Completeness of revascularization
5. Intraoperative myocardial protection.
6. Suitability of the coronary vessels for bypass
7. Surgical skill
8. Peri-operative injury
9. Graft closure or restenosis
10. Associated primary cardiomyopathy
11. Left ventricular dilatation

An improvement in LV function after coronary revascularization depends on the ability to reliably detect changes in LV function. This assessment has been based on analyses of wall motion and EF, which are done either with two-dimensional echocardiography or with gated blood pool imaging (MUGA). More sophisticated techniques, such as quantitative assessment based on the centerline method available with contrast ventriculography, magnetic resonance imaging, two-dimensional echocardiography, and MUGA, are often not used. Analysis of wall motion is most commonly performed based on subjective assessment. This type of analysis is rather primitive when compared to the sophisticated technologies that are used to detect the presence or absence of viable myocardium. It is conceivable that, in the future, three-dimensional tomographic MUGA studies or three-dimensional echocardiographic studies with quantitative assessment of regional and global LV function will provide more rewarding results. It should also be noted that assessment of the septal wall motion may be difficult after surgery because wall motion abnormality commonly occurs after surgery. Such abnormality may exist even though the septum is 'viable' and the myocardial blood flow is normal. This type of motion abnormality may persist for as long as 6 months after surgery but is often mild and does not have a major impact on EF.

The timing of EF measurement is also important. Early assessment after surgery may underestimate the improvement, possibly because of residual myocardial stunning. Assessment at 6–8 weeks is probably preferable. We examined the EF by MUGA early (6 ± 4 days) and late (62 ± 24 days) after surgery in two groups of patients. Those with normal pre-operative EF (Group 1, $n = 12$) and those with LV dysfunction (Group 2, $n = 15$). Group 1 showed no significant change in EF: pre-operative, 62%; early post-operative, 64%; and late post-operative, 63%. In Group 2, however, the EF improved more in the late studies than the early studies. Thus, the EF was 26 ± 8% pre-operatively, 30 ± 10% early after CABG, and 34 ± 8% late after CABG (P <0.05). There was improvement of 5% or more in EF in 4 patients early but in 11 patients late after surgery (P <0.05). Although the patients who had early improvement continued to show such improvement in the late study, additionally, 7 patients only showed improvement in the late study. Thus, the timing of measurement is important in patients with LV dysfunction; early assessment may underestimate the prevalence and degree of recovery. In patients undergoing percutaneous transluminal coronary angioplasty, the timing is also important but there are different confounding factors. For example, measurement 8–12 weeks after the intervention may not show improvement because of restenosis which occurs in 40–50% of patients. Therefore, in such patients, early assessment (1–2 weeks) appears to be more appropriate.

It should also be mentioned that, to be clinically meaningful, the change in EF should not only be statistically significant but clinically relevant. For example, a change from 22% to 25% may be statistically significant but is hardly clinically relevant. Similarly, a slight improvement in wall motion may be statistically significant but clinically irrelevant. For interventions to affect the quality of life and prognosis, improvement in EF should be the goal of intervention.

Improvement in EF must necessarily depend on the extent of the viable hibernating myocardium. Therefore, quantitative assessment is important. Improvement is probably unlikely if the extent is <20% of the myocardium.

The extent of viable myocardium is important in determining the degree of improvement in LV function after coronary revascularization. The presence of a small area of viable myocardium in a patient with severe dysfunction may be insufficient to improve LV function post-operatively; therefore, the detection of viability, is not in itself an indication for coronary revascularization. Not only should the extent of viable hibernating myocardium be large enough but the coronary anatomy should be suitable. The suitability of the coronary anatomy underscores the central role of coronary angiography in selecting candidates for revascularization. For example, poor run-off due to severe diffuse disease in the left anterior descending artery is unlikely to result in regional and global improvement after revascularization, despite the presence of viable myocardium in the territory of this vessel, and regardless of patency and number of grafts to the remaining vessels. Obviously, if the patient suffers a peri-operative necrosis the beneficial effect of revascularization will be negated. It is important to keep in mind that peri-operative necrosis cannot always be diagnosed on clinical grounds and by electrocardiographic or enzymatic changes [26,27].

Another important factor that should be considered is the presence of unrelated primary cardiomyopathy [12]. Single-photon perfusion images, myocardial blood flow, and metabolic studies suggest that patients with primary cardiomyopathy have normal or near-normal studies and, therefore, these patients will be considered to have 'viable' myocardium; the LV dysfunction which is not due to myocardial ischemia. The usual clinical scenario is a patient with severe LV dysfunction which is out of proportion to the severity and extent of CAD. It is quite possible, therefore, that such patients may have two unrelated disease entities and coronary revascularization will not result in improvement in LV function.

LV size is probably also an important determinant of recovery of function; patients with marked LV dilation probably do not show improvement. The perfusion images of patients who show improvement in LV function after revascularization often indicate that these patients do not have marked LV dilation. The LV dilation is due to both infarct expansion and remodeling, therefore, even myocardial segments with normal perfusion may have systolic dysfunction. The degree of LV dilation beyond which recovery of LV function is unusual is unclear and, therefore, it is important that future studies should include quantitative measurement of LV volume in addition to assessment of EF and wall motion.

Conclusions

We have powerful tools for the assessment of viable myocardium in patients with LV dysfunction. Patients with viable myocardium due to hibernation/stunning are likely to show improvement in contractile function after coronary revascularization. Depending on several factors, the degree of improvement may be considerable. Associated with improvement is increased survival and improvement in symptoms of congestive heart failure. Indications for revascularization in such patients is primarily to improve prognosis and symptoms of congestive heart failure. In patients who have symptoms related to ischemia, i.e. angina pectoris, coronary revascularization is predominantly indicated for alleviation of symptoms. In patients with LV dysfunction due to scarring, i.e. nonviable myocardium, coronary revascularization not only carries a high risk but does not result in improvement in symptoms or prognosis; therefore, the judicial use of coronary revascularization appears to be cost-effective in properly selected patients.

The choice of the diagnostic technique depends on expertise and available resources. Single-photon imaging is probably widely available. Positron emission tomography, magnetic resonance imaging, and contrast echocardiography are important tools but may be limited by cost (positron emission tomography and magnetic resonance imaging) or by the need of cardiac catheterization and intracoronary administration (contrast echocardiography).

It should be noted that patients who require viability studies, as defined in this book, are those with severe LV dysfunction either on a global or regional basis. Therefore, patients who have preserved wall motion are not candidates for viability studies because, by definition, these patients have viable myocardium. Similarly, patients with preserved wall thickening have viable myocardium. It is in patients in whom wall motion or thickening is abnormal or unknown that viability studies are important. These areas could be regional, as in the case in post-infarction patients, or global, as in patients with depressed EF. Since patients with hibernation have reduced coronary blood flow at rest, it is quite conceivable that dobutamine infusion or any other inotropic intervention may not improve the function in such segments. On the contrary, they may produce deterioration if they result in an increase in myocardial oxygen demand. A transient improvement may, however, be due to inotropic stimulation that is uncoupled for changes in myocardial blood flow. Therefore, the lack of improvement with any one of these interventions may not be sufficient to exclude the possibility of viable myocardium. An acceptable accoustic window may not be present in many patients and the interpretation is subjective. The technique, however, may be an acceptable alternative in centers where high quality nuclear techniques are unavailable.

On the other hand, scintigraphic techniques appear to be the procedures of choice as they not only allow detection but also quantification of the extent of the viable myocardium. Nevertheless, partial volume effect due to lack of myocardial thickening may potentially be a reason why some segments that are classified as nonviable by imaging show improvement after coronary revascularization. In the future, attenuation correction methods may eliminate some of the artifacts that contribute to misinterpretation. Attenuation correction may explain why positron emission tomography is superior to single-photon imaging in addressing viability in the inferior wall, while these two imaging modalities are comparable in assessing viability in the territory of the left anterior descending artery. Finally, the role of labeled fatty acid imaging needs to be addressed in the future but, both our initial experience and more recent studies suggesting the superior role of oxidative metabolism in assessing myocardial viability by positron emission tomography, would indicate a definite role.

References

1. Iskandrian AS, Verani MS. Myocardial Viability in Nuclear Cardiac Imaging: Principles and Applications. 2nd ed. Philadelphia: FA Davis Publishers. In press.
2. Iskandrian AS, Heo J, Nguyen T. Current and emerging scintigraphic methods to assess myocardial viability and their clinical importance. Am J Card Imaging 1992; 6: 16–27.
3. Iskandrian AS, Heo J, Helfant RH, Segal BL. Chronic myocardial ischemia and left ventricular function. Ann Intern Med 1987; 107: 925–7.
4. Lemlek J, Heo J, Iskandrian AS. The clinical relevance of myocardial viability in patient management. Am Heart J 1992; 124: 1327–31.
5. Rahimtoola SH. A perspective on the three large multicenter randomized clinical trials of coronary bypass surgery for chronic stable angina. Circulation 1985; 72: V123–35.

6. Schelbert HR, Buxton D. Insights into coronary artery disease gained from metabolic imaging. Circulation 1988; 78: 496–505.

7. Rahimtoola SH. Coronary bypass surgery for chronic angina – 1981. A perspective. Circulation 1982; 65: 225–41.

8. Braunwald E, Rutherford JD. Reversible ischemic left ventricular dysfunction: Evidence for the 'hibernating myocardium'. J Am Coll Cardiol 1986; 8: 1467–70.

9. Sabia PJ, Powers ER, Ragosta M, Sarembock IJ, Burwell LR, Kaul S. An association between collateral blood flow and myocardial viability in patients with recent myocardial infarction. N Engl J Med 1992; 327: 1825–31.

10. Dilsizian V, Rocco TP, Freedman NM, Leon MB, Bonow RO. Enhanced detection of ischemic but viable myocardium by the reinjection of thallium after stress-redistribution imaging. N Engl J Med 1990; 323: 141–6.

11. Iskandrian AS, Hakki AH, Kane SA, Goel IP, Mundth ED, Segal BL. Rest and redistribution thallium-201 myocardial scintigraphy to predict improvement in left ventricular function after coronary arterial bypass grafting. Am J Cardiol 1983; 51: 1312–6.

12. Iskandrian AS, Helfeld H, Lemlek J, Lee J, Iskandrian B, Heo J. Differentiation between primary dilated cardiomyopathy and ischemic cardiomyopathy based on right ventricular performance. Am Heart J 1992; 123: 768–73.

13. Tillisch J, Brunker R, Marshall R, Schwaiger M, Mandelkern M, Phelps M *et al*. Reversibility of cardiac wall motion abnormalities predicted by positron tomography. N Engl J Med 1986; 314: 884–8.

14. Wolmer I, Powers J, Sung KK, Cave V, Wasserleben V, Cassel D *et al*. Detection of myocardial viability using dynamic SPECT I-123-IPPA imaging [abstract]. Circulation 1993; 88 (4 Suppl I): I200.

15. Fragasso G, Margonato A, Chierchia SL. Assessment of viability after myocardial infarction: Clinical relevance and methodological problems. Int J Card Imaging 1993; 9 (Suppl 1): 3–10.

16. Rozanski A, Berman DS, Gray R, Levy R, Raymond M, Maddahi J *et al*. Use of thallium-201 redistribution scintigraphy in the preoperative differentiation of reversible and nonreversible myocardial asynergy. Circulation 1981; 64: 936–44.

17. Gibson RS, Watson DD, Taylor GJ, Crosby IK, Wellons HL, Holt ND *et al*. Prospective assessment of regional myocardial perfusion before and after coronary revascularization surgery by quantitative thallium-201 scintigraphy. J Am Coll Cardiol 1983; 1: 804–15.

18. Tamaki N, Yonekura Y, Yamashita K, Mukai T, Magata Y, Hashimoto T *et al*. SPECT thallium 201 tomography and positron tomography using N-13 ammonia and F-18 fluorodeoxyglucose in coronary heart disease. Am J Card Imaging 1989; 3: 3–9.

19. Gropler RJ, Geltman EM, Sampathkumaran K, Perez JE, Schechtman KB, Conversano A *et al*. Comparison of Carbon-11-acetate with fluorine-18-fluorodeoxyglucose for delineating viable myocardium by positron emission tomography. J Am Coll Cardiol 1993; 22: 1587–97.

20. Aksut S, Wolmer I, Pancholy S, Mallavarapu C, Heo J, Iskandrian AS. Rest-redistribution SPECT thallium imaging to assess viability in patients with left ventricular dysfunction [abstract]. J Nucl Med 1993; 34 (5 Suppl): 85P.

21. Dilsizian V, Bonow RO. Current diagnostic techniques of assessing myocardial viability in patients with hibernating and stunned myocardium. Circulation 1993; 87: 1–20.

22. Ragosta M, Beller GA, Watson DD, Kaul S, Gimple LW. Quantitative planar rest-redistribution 201Tl imaging in detection of myocardial viability and prediction of improvement in left ventricular function after coronary bypass surgery in patients with severely depressed left ventricular function. Circulation 1993; 87: 1630–41.

23. Dilzisian V, Perrone-Filardi P, Arrighi JA, Bacharach SL, Quyyumi AA, Freedman NMT *et al*. Concordance and discordance between stress-redistribution-reinjection and rest-redistribution thallium imaging for assessing viable myocardium. Circulation 1993; 88: 941–52.

24. Van Eck-Smit BLF, van der Wall EE, Kuiper AFM, Zwinderman AH, Pauwels EKJ. Immediate thallium-201 reinjection following stress imaging: A time-saving approach for detection of myocardial viability. J Nucl Med 1993; 34: 737–43.

25. Kuijper AFM, Vliegen HW, van der Wall EE, Oosterhuis WP, Zwinderman AH, van Eck-Smit

BLF *et al.* The clinical impact of thallium-201 reinjection scintigraphy for detection of myocardial viability. Eur J Nucl Med 1992; 19: 783–9.

26. Mahmarian JJ, Pratt EM, Borges-Neto S, Cashion WR, Roberts R, Verani MS. Quantification of infarct size by 201Tl single-photon emission computed tomography during acute myocardial infarction in humans. Comparison with enzymatic estimates. Circulation 1988; 78: 831–9.

27. Iskandrian AS, Kegel JG, Tecce MA, Wasserleben V, Cave V, Heo J. Simultaneous assessment of left ventricular perfusion and function with technetium-99m sestamibi after coronary artery bypass grafting. Am Heart J 1993; 126: 1199–203.

Index

Developments in Cardiovascular Medicine

1. Ch.T. Lancée (ed.): *Echocardiology.* 1979   ISBN 90-247-2209-8
2. J. Baan, A.C. Arntzenius and E.L. Yellin (eds.): *Cardiac Dynamics.* 1980
   ISBN 90-247-2212-8
3. H.J.Th. Thalen and C.C. Meere (eds.): *Fundamentals of Cardiac Pacing.* 1979
   ISBN 90-247-2245-4
4. H.E. Kulbertus and H.J.J. Wellens (eds.): *Sudden Death.* 1980   ISBN 90-247-2290-X
5. L.S. Dreifus and A.N. Brest (eds.): *Clinical Applications of Cardiovascular Drugs.*
   1980   ISBN 90-247-2295-0
6. M.P. Spencer and J.M. Reid: *Cerebrovascular Evaluation with Doppler Ultrasound.*
   With contributions by E.C. Brockenbrough, R.S. Reneman, G.I. Thomas and D.L.
   Davis. 1981   ISBN 90-247-2384-1
7. D.P. Zipes, J.C. Bailey and V. Elharrar (eds.): *The Slow Inward Current and Cardiac
   Arrhythmias.* 1980   ISBN 90-247-2380-9
8. H. Kesteloot and J.V. Joossens (eds.): *Epidemiology of Arterial Blood Pressure.* 1980
   ISBN 90-247-2386-8
9. F.J.Th. Wackers (ed.): *Thallium-201 and Technetium-99m-Pyrophosphate. Myocardial Imaging in the Coronary Care Unit.* 1980   ISBN 90-247-2396-5
10. A. Maseri, C. Marchesi, S. Chierchia and M.G. Trivella (eds.): *Coronary Care Units.*
    Proceedings of a European Seminar (1978). 1981   ISBN 90-247-2456-2
11. J. Morganroth, E.N. Moore, L.S. Dreifus and E.L. Michelson (eds.): *The Evaluation of
    New Antiarrhythmic Drugs.* Proceedings of the First Symposium on New Drugs and
    Devices, held in Philadelphia, Pa., U.S.A. (1980). 1981   ISBN 90-247-2474-0
12. P. Alboni: *Intraventricular Conduction Disturbances.* 1981   ISBN 90-247-2483-X
13. H. Rijsterborgh (ed.): *Echocardiology.* 1981   ISBN 90-247-2491-0
14. G.S. Wagner (ed.): *Myocardial Infarction.* Measurement and Intervention. 1982
    ISBN 90-247-2513-5
15. R.S. Meltzer and J. Roelandt (eds.): *Contrast Echocardiography.* 1982
    ISBN 90-247-2531-3
16. A. Amery, R. Fagard, P. Lijnen and J. Staessen (eds.): *Hypertensive Cardiovascular
    Disease.* Pathophysiology and Treatment. 1982   IBSN 90-247-2534-8
17. L.N. Bouman and H.J. Jongsma (eds.): *Cardiac Rate and Rhythm.* Physiological,
    Morphological and Developmental Aspects. 1982   ISBN 90-247-2626-3
18. J. Morganroth and E.N. Moore (eds.): *The Evaluation of Beta Blocker and Calcium
    Antagonist Drugs.* Proceedings of the 2nd Symposium on New Drugs and Devices,
    held in Philadelphia, Pa., U.S.A. (1981). 1982   ISBN 90-247-2642-5
19. M.B. Rosenbaum and M.V. Elizari (eds.): *Frontiers of Cardiac Electrophysiology.*
    1983   ISBN 90-247-2663-8
20. J. Roelandt and P.G. Hugenholtz (eds.): *Long-term Ambulatory Electrocardiography.*
    1982   ISBN 90-247-2664-6
21. A.A.J. Adgey (ed.): *Acute Phase of Ischemic Heart Disease and Myocardial Infarc-
    tion.* 1982   ISBN 90-247-2675-1
22. P. Hanrath, W. Bleifeld and J. Souquet (eds.): *Cardiovascular Diagnosis by Ultra-
    sound.* Transesophageal, Computerized, Contrast, Doppler Echocardiography. 1982
    ISBN 90-247-2692-1
23. J. Roelandt (ed.): *The Practice of M-Mode and Two-dimensional Echocardiography.*
    1983   ISBN 90-247-2745-6
24. J. Meyer, P. Schweizer and R. Erbel (eds.): *Advances in Noninvasive Cardiology.*
    Ultrasound, Computed Tomography, Radioisotopes, Digital Angiography. 1983
    ISBN 0-89838-576-8
25. J. Morganroth and E.N. Moore (eds.): *Sudden Cardiac Death and Congestive Heart
    Failure.* Diagnosis and Treatment. Proceedings of the 3rd Symposium on New Drugs
    and Devices, held in Philadelphia, Pa., U.S.A. (1982). 1983   ISBN 0-89838-580-6
26. H.M. Perry Jr. (ed.): *Lifelong Management of Hypertension.* 1983
    ISBN 0-89838-582-2
27. E.A. Jaffe (ed.): *Biology of Endothelial Cells.* 1984   ISBN 0-89838-587-3

Developments in Cardiovascular Medicine

Developments in Cardiovascular Medicine

Developments in Cardiovascular Medicine

Developments in Cardiovascular Medicine

Developments in Cardiovascular Medicine

121. S. Sideman, R. Beyar and A.G. Kleber (eds.): *Cardiac Electrophysiology, Circulation, and Transport.* Proceedings of the 7th Henry Goldberg Workshop (Berne, Switzerland, 1990). 1991   ISBN 0-7923-1145-0
122. D.M. Bers: *Excitation-Contraction Coupling and Cardiac Contractile Force.* 1991
                                                                                 ISBN 0-7923-1186-8
123. A.-M. Salmasi and A.N. Nicolaides (eds.): *Occult Atherosclerotic Disease.* Diagnosis, Assessment and Management. 1991   ISBN 0-7923-1188-4
124. J.A.E. Spaan: *Coronary Blood Flow.* Mechanics, Distribution, and Control. 1991
                                                                                 ISBN 0-7923-1210-4
125. R.W. Stout (ed.): *Diabetes and Atherosclerosis.* 1991   ISBN 0-7923-1310-0
126. A.G. Herman (ed.): *Antithrombotics.* Pathophysiological Rationale for Pharmacological Interventions. 1991   ISBN 0-7923-1413-1
127. N.H.J. Pijls: *Maximal Myocardial Perfusion as a Measure of the Functional Significance of Coronary Arteriogram.* From a Pathoanatomic to a Pathophysiologic Interpretation of the Coronary Arteriogram. 1991   ISBN 0-7923-1430-1
128. J.H.C. Reiber and E.E. v.d. Wall (eds.): *Cardiovascular Nuclear Medicine and MRI.* Quantitation and Clinical Applications. 1992   ISBN 0-7923-1467-0
129. E. Andries, P. Brugada and R. Stroobrandt (eds.): *How to Face 'the Faces' of Cardiac Pacing.* 1992   ISBN 0-7923-1528-6
130. M. Nagano, S. Mochizuki and N.S. Dhalla (eds.): *Cardiovascular Disease in Diabetes.* 1992   ISBN 0-7923-1554-5
131. P.W. Serruys, B.H. Strauss and S.B. King III (eds.): *Restenosis after Intervention with New Mechanical Devices.* 1992   ISBN 0-7923-1555-3
132. P.J. Walter (ed.): *Quality of Life after Open Heart Surgery.* 1992
                                                                                 ISBN 0-7923-1580-4
133. E.E. van der Wall, H. Sochor, A. Righetti and M.G. Niemeyer (eds.): *What's new in Cardiac Imaging?* SPECT, PET and MRI. 1992   ISBN 0-7923-1615-0
134. P. Hanrath, R. Uebis and W. Krebs (eds.): *Cardiovascular Imaging by Ultrasound.* 1992   ISBN 0-7923-1755-6
135. F.H. Messerli (ed.): *Cardiovascular Disease in the Elderly.* 3rd ed. 1992
                                                                                 ISBN 0-7923-1859-5
136. J. Hess and G.R. Sutherland (eds.): *Congenital Heart Disease in Adolescents and Adults.* 1992   ISBN 0-7923-1862-5
137. J.H.C. Reiber and P.W. Serruys (eds.): *Advances in Quantitative Coronary Arteriography.* 1993   ISBN 0-7923-1863-3
138. A.-M. Salmasi and A.S. Iskandrian (eds.): *Cardiac Output and Regional Flow in Health and Disease.* 1993   ISBN 0-7923-1911-7
139. J.H. Kingma, N.M. van Hemel and K.I. Lie (eds.): *Atrial Fibrillation, a Treatable Disease?* 1992   ISBN 0-7923-2008-5
140. B. Ostadel and N.S. Dhalla (eds.): *Heart Function in Health and Disease.* Proceedings of the Cardiovascular Program (Prague, Czechoslovakia, 1991). 1992
                                                                                 ISBN 0-7923-2052-2
141. D. Noble and Y.E. Earm (eds.): *Ionic Channels and Effect of Taurine on the Heart.* Proceedings of an International Symposium (Seoul, Korea, 1992). 1993
                                                                                 ISBN 0-7923-2199-5
142. H.M. Piper and C.J. Preusse (eds.): *Ischemia-reperfusion in Cardiac Surgery.* 1993
                                                                                 ISBN 0-7923-2241-X
143. J. Roelandt, E.J. Gussenhoven and N. Bom (eds.): *Intravascular Ultrasound.* 1993
                                                                                 ISBN 0-7923-2301-7
144. M.E. Safar and M.F. O'Rourke (eds.): *The Arterial System in Hypertension.* 1993
                                                                                 ISBN 0-7923-2343-2
145. P.W. Serruys, D.P. Foley and P.J. de Feyter (eds.): *Quantitative Coronary Angiography in Clinical Practice.* With a Foreword by Spencer B. King III. 1994
                                                                                 ISBN 0-7923-2368-8

Developments in Cardiovascular Medicine

Previous volumes are still available

KLUWER ACADEMIC PUBLISHERS – DORDRECHT / BOSTON / LONDON

Made in the USA
Las Vegas, NV
11 August 2022

53087764R00120